THE ESSENTIAL OIL TRUTH

the facts without the hype

Renee V. Keilman
(520) 404-8277
YoungLiving.org/2Suns2thFairy

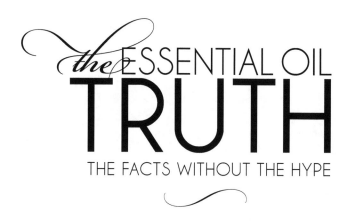

the ESSENTIAL OIL
TRUTH

THE FACTS WITHOUT THE HYPE

SECOND EDITION

JEN O'SULLIVAN

The Essential Oil Truth: the Facts Without the Hype
Copyright © 2015 by Jen O'Sullivan
www.JenEssentials.com

Cover Design and Photography by Jen O'Sullivan
Interior Photography by Jen O'Sullivan

ISBN: 978-153-347430-8

First Printing, 2015.
Second Edition, May 2016.
Create Space Publishing

Printed in the United States of America

May 2016

10 9 8 7 6 5 4 3 2

It is with much gratitude that I say, "thank you" to my essential oil family for helping me make this book a reality. Thank you, Jessica Petty, for encouraging me to share my love of essential oils with the world and to become "The Oil Lady." I am truly indebted to Jade Shutes and Cathy Skipper at The School for Aromatic Studies for the educational care they provided me. Thank you, Jacob O'Sullivan, my incredible helper and son who is always ready to get oiled up and try new adventures with me. And, thank you to my amazing husband, Tim O'Sullivan for supporting me through the months of writing, all the while, cheering me on, straight through the finish line. You are my true blessing in this life! Without all of their help & support this book would not be in your hands.

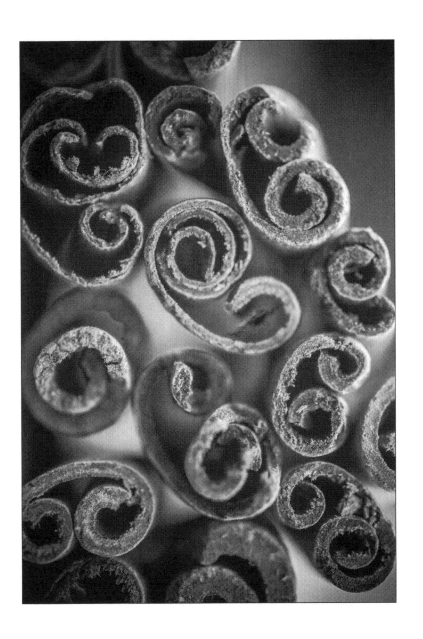

CONTENTS

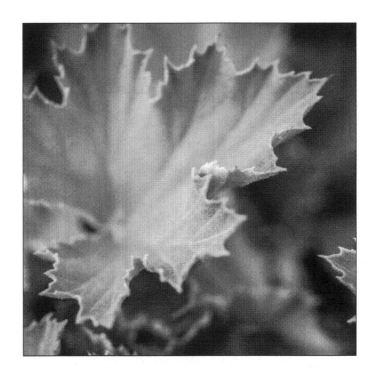

"TOO MANY OF US CONSIDER PEOPLE WITH

TITLES

OR A LONG LIST OF CREDENTIALS

trustworthy

ONLY TO FIND OUT THEY WERE

WRONG."

TheEssentialOilTruth.com

PREFACE

A NOTE FROM THE AUTHOR

I am a skeptic… a BIG one. I don't trust many people and I honestly think there is so much out there that is passed off as "fact" when it may not be. Just because it is published on a web page, written in a book, televised on a newscast, or even spouted from the lips of our trusted doctors, does not mean it is the exact truth. Too many of us consider certain people with titles or a long list of credentials trustworthy, only to find out they were wrong.

So, why listen to me? I am certified in French Medicinal Aromatherapy from The School for Aromatic Studies, and have been educating people about essential oil use since 2007. I have been a college professor for 13 years, a high school teacher for 14 years, have owned an educational small business marketing and coaching corporation for five years, and have published four books, two on business and two on education.

My friends, family, and colleagues know me as a hound dog for research. If they can't figure something out, they will often ask me. I have always been someone who, when told something that is suspect by someone else with seemingly trustworthy passion, still will not believe what they say until I've found three other reputable sources that validate their passionate statement. I think it stems from my childhood. My older sister used to trick and prank me to no end. So much so, that as a child, I was labeled "the gullible one." Fun for her, not so much for me.

After I wised up somewhere around my tweens, I decided to be THAT person. You know, the person who studies, researches, and works it until it cannot be worked anymore. I was the person in college that everyone came to for notes when they missed class. I am now the person that people come to when they are really in a bind because they know I usually have answers.

The issue for me, when it comes to essential oils, is that everything I hear seems to always be one-sided, usually with a major slant toward one specific brand. I wanted to come at it from a neutral perspective. I do realize there are some things that will not be neutral, but I have studied both of the major opposing essential oil experts, Dr. David Stewart and Robert Tisserand, along with other experts, and I was able to cross reference a lot of what they teach through colleges and resources in Europe that do not have a monetary stake in a particular essential oil company.

My main concern has always been the major hearsay that surrounds essential oils. There are some things you will read from several authors who are experts on the subject that simply cannot be verified through any available source, so those items I have left out. Again, my goal is to give you the facts without the hype. All in all, I have tried really hard to stick to only the facts.

As for my essential oil background, I was on a mission to figure out how to properly bring a new human being into the world. I was convinced that the chemical-laden, toxic environment we have created for ourselves was not conducive to this new little human we desired to create. So I did my research. I researched all the chemical-free cleaners and products, went vegan, and studied nutrition and overall home health for several months, which then turned into a life-long love affair with health and wellness. I took multiple classes, seminars, and workshops on nutrition, gut issues, and how the things we ingest, breathe in, and place on our bodies affects our whole-body and life health and wellness.

I devoured nutrition books such as *The China Study, Excitotoxins, The Taste that Kills, Skinny Bitch* (it is like *The China Study* easy version), *Wheat Belly,* and all sorts of movies and documentaries that I am sure you all have seen such as *Forks Over Knives, Food Inc., Super Size Me, Fat Sick and Nearly Dead*. Honestly, if it was on nutrition, I watched it.

I got heavily into whole food nutrition right alongside my meat-eating, fast-food-grubbing husband who still, to this day, goes and fills up on things I personally would never consume. But there you have it. We are all on our own path. You won't find any judgment here. To give you a little about who I am outside of my passion for research and understanding, here are some fun facts:

I am a total Jesus lover who will always give Him credit for any accomplishments, small or large. I love my husband the most on this earth. I love my son a close second and he knows it, but wouldn't have it any other way. I am the girl that hates the gym and would much rather be outside. I am a competitive cyclist, avid snowboarder, commercial and private photographer, web designer, graphic designer, book binder, author, business and life coach, health and wellness advocate, high school teacher and college professor, event producer, marketing director, entrepreneur, domain name hoarder (is there such a thing?), blogger, vlogger (YouTube video blogger), flogger (Facebook blogger), Periscope addict, and pianist. I know, all sort of random but aren't we all sort of random? That is what is so great about life!

My reason for writing this book is simply because when I got into essential oils I found that there was a lot of misinformation, speculation and assumption going around, as well as a lot of bad advice given by people who never did their research. My hope is to dispel some of the myths and rumors about essential oils, and that my countless hours through the years of reading, researching, and instruction will help you gain a greater understanding of the true nature and beauty of essential oils and their proper use for your everyday health and well-being.

~ Jen O'Sullivan

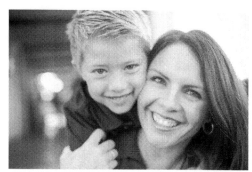

Me and my son, Jacob. Photo credit: Max Garabedian.

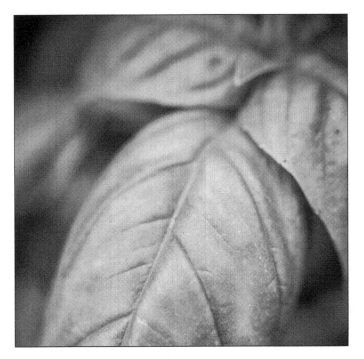

" THEIR FRUIT WILL BE FOR FOOD, AND THEIR

LEAVES

FOR *healing*. "

TheEssentialOilTruth.com

EZEKIEL 47:12 (ESV)

INTRODUCTION

THE VERY BASICS OF ESSENTIAL OILS

What are essential oils?
Essential oils are the life-force of the plant, much like our blood.

How do you use them?
You use them topically, aromatically, or internally (only internal when stated on the label as a dietary supplement).

How do they work?
Just like our blood helps to oxygenate, regulate, and heal our bodies; essential oils do the same for the plant source they are extracted from. They help support and regulate our body systems.

Who should use them?
Everyone should use them; animals and humans alike.

Why should we use them?
They help raise the health of our body functions to support proper health and wellness.

When should we use them?
Every day and often. Essential oils are not single-use fixes. They should be looked at like any other wellness regime we embark upon. You don't start and stop a diet in one day (OK, some of us do) but when you want results and overall wellness, you do something long-term, as you should with essential oils.

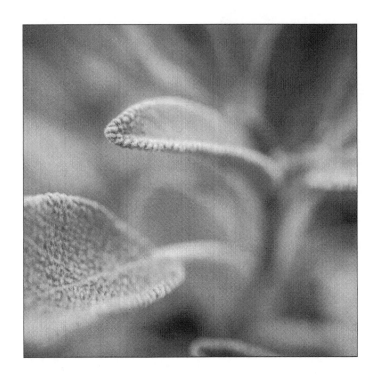

"ESSENTIAL OILS ARE THE

life force

of plants."

48 LESSONS

ALL YOU NEED TO KNOW IN 48 MICRO LESSONS

Lesson #1

WHAT EXACTLY ARE ESSENTIAL OILS?

Essential oils are the life-force of plants; basically their internal juices. The essential oil is to a plant as blood is to a human. The juices are called the Oleo-Resin-Gum part of the plant. The oleo is the lipid-soluble and volatile part of the plant juices, and what mostly make up essential oils. Resin is the alcohol-soluble part. Gum is the water-soluble part.

The word "oleo" is where we get the term "essential oils" because the oleo part is the volatile part of the plant juice. Rather than call it "oleo," which is derived from the Latin word "oleum" for oil, the term "essential oil" is what we call it today. Volatile means a substance's ability to leap into the air. It is why all essential oils are fragrant and why you are able to smell some of the more potent oils from across the room just by opening the bottle.

They are composed of three major fractions called phenols, monoterpenes, and sesquiterpenes. There are many different types of essential oils based on how they were produced from cultivation to distillation, and finding out which type is right for you is exactly what this book is about.

Lesson #2
THE HISTORY OF ESSENTIAL OILS

The historical use of essential oils dates back to Egyptian hieroglyphics that were drawn over 5000 years ago. Here are some fun facts about essential oils throughout history:

• Circa 5000 BC: Anthropological evidence found of aromatic plant life used with olive and sesame oils to create ointments.

• 3200 BC: Egyptians used resins such as Frankincense and Myrrh as part of their embalming process.

• 3000 BC: The first primitive still was discovered in 1975 in Indus Valley Civilization during the Bronze Age, which dates back to 3000 BC.

• 1300s BC: King Tut's tomb contained alabaster jars filled with Frankincense essential oil.

• 400 BC: Hippocrates, a Greek physician used essential oils in his treatments.

• 100 BC: There are reports of Rome consuming 2800 tons of Frankincense and 500 tons of Myrrh per year.

• Circa 1600 BC to 85 AD: The Old and New Testament has hundreds of references to the use of essential oils.

• 1340 AD: The Bubonic Plague was underway and apothecaries (like our modern day pharmacists) figured out how to rub their bodies with a recipe of essential oils in order to rob the dead of their belongings and not contract the deadly plague. Legend states that officials lessened their sentence of death if they gave up their recipe.

• 1910: Dr. Rene Gattefosse (French chemist) severely burned his arm and used Lavender essential oil as a last resort. To his surprise his burn healed without any scarring. He went on to coin the term Aromatherapy in the 1920s.

• 1964: Dr. Jean Balnet published "The Practice of Aromatherapy." He found long-term psychiatric patients were greatly helped after he administered essential oils.

• 1974: R. Deininger conducted a double-blind study on essential oils and the autonomic nervous system. He proved the effectiveness of essential oils in balancing the nervous system.

Lesson #3

FROM CHEMISTS, DOCTORS, & AROMATHERAPISTS

"The present study confirmed that the essential oils and organic extracts of the Sicilian rosemary samples analyzed showed a considerable antioxidant/free radical-scavenging activity." Napoli EM, Et al., Istituto del C.N.R. di Chimica Biomolecolare, Via Paolo Gaifami, 2015

"Using cancer cell apoptosis induction trials, previous studies have identified that specific components of myrrh and frankincense essential oils are capable of inducing cancer cell apoptosis. For example, sesquiterpenes have anticancer activities that are likely to arrest the proliferation of prostate cancer cells in the G0/G1 phase." Yingli Chen, Et al., College of Pharmacy, Harbin Medical University-Daquin, China 2013

"Every educated physician knows that most diseases are not appreciably helped by medicine." Richard C. Cabot, M.D. Professor Harvard School of Medicine; Author of *Differential Diagnosis, The Art of Ministering to the Sick*

"Drugs and oils work in opposite ways. Drugs toxify. Oils detoxify. Drugs clog and confuse receptor sites. Oils clean receptor sites. Drugs depress the immune system. Oils strengthen the immune system. Antibiotics attack bacteria indiscriminately, killing both the good and the bad. Oils attack only the harmful bacteria, allowing our body's friendly flora to flourish." David Stewart, Ph.D., R.A., *The Chemistry of Essential Oils*, 2005

"Boswellia sacra [Sacred Frankincense from Oman and Yemen] essential oil induces breast cancer cell-specific cytotoxicity. Suppression of cellular network formation and disruption of spheroid development of breast cancer cells by Boswellia sacra essential oil suggest that the essential oil may be effective for advanced breast cancer. Consistently, the essential oil represses signaling pathways and cell cycle regulators that have been proposed as therapeutic targets for breast cancer." Mahmoud M Suhail, et al., Al Afia Medical Complex, Salalah, Sultanate of Oman, 2011

"Our bodies are biologically programmed to react to essential oil constituents, which interact with a variety of receptor sites, neurochemicals and enzymes, giving them a potential for therapeutic activity."
Robert Tisserand

"Essential oils promote natural healing by stimulating and reinforcing the body's own mechanisms. Essences of chamomile and thyme, for instance, are credited with the ability to stimulate the production of white blood cells which help in our fight against disease." Chrissie Wildwood, 1991

"Essential oils include muscle relaxants, digestive tonics, circulatory stimulants and hormone precursors. Many repair injured cells; others carry away metabolic waste. In addition, a number of essential oils enhance immunity, working with the body to heal itself. They're capable of stimulating the production of phagocytes (white blood cells that attack invaders)." Keville and Green, 1995

"What do the oils do? First of all they are transporters; they transport products to the cells of our body. Secondly, they contain ATP, which serves as the power source of the cells–the fuel. Essential oils normalize the viscosity of the blood, and facilitate the delivery of vital nutrients. Others release liver toxins, clean the gall bladder, and stimulate the secretion of gastric juices, while even others work to improve nerve impulses and synaptic connections." Friedmann, 1995

"Essential oils are the regenerating and oxygenating immune defense properties of plants. Their oxygenating molecules effectively transport nutrients and a myriad of other powerful chemical constituents to the cells, bringing life to the plants, destroying infections, staving off infestation, aiding in growth, and stimulating healing. They are to plants what blood is to the human body, and much, much more."
D. Gary Young, ND, 1995

"Certain aldehydes in lemon balm, for instance, have been shown to reduce inflammation, while certain ketones in rosemary and eucalyptus appear to reduce mucus production. Essential oils appear to affect the emotions as well: In one recent study done in a British nursing home, vaporized lavender oil was found to work as well as pharmaceutical sedatives in helping residents relax into sleep." Dr. Andrew Weil, 1996

Lesson #4
HOW & WHY ESSENTIAL OILS WORK

The human body is composed of around 100 trillion cells. Essential oils are composed of around 40 million trillion molecules per single drop! That is 40,000,000,000,000,000,000. Can you even fathom that number? Why and how can that many molecules fit into one single drop of essential oil? Simple; their molecules are extraordinarily small. They are all less than 300 Daltons or amu (atomic mass units) in weight.

Why this matters to us is that they are able to pass through all of our tissues and directly into our cells. The body's transportation system is extremely effective and can transport these molecules all over the body within minutes when placed anywhere on the body. By simply placing a drop of Peppermint essential oil on the bottom of your feet, in 20 minutes your entire body will be infiltrated with 40 million trillion molecules, in effect consuming every cell in your body with 400,000 molecules each! Astounding.

Let's look at two areas that are somewhat controversial in the world of essential oil use: the blood brain barrier and cancer.

The blood brain barrier is a touchy subject for some, simply because we understand it to be our protection from allowing harmful substances into the part of our body that makes you, you. We know that brain cancer is untreatable with chemotherapy, simply because the majority of the molecules found in chemotherapy treatment are larger than the filter on the blood brain barrier.

It is understood that in order to cross the blood brain barrier a molecule needs to be less than 1,000 to 800 Daltons and some are now saying it is under 400 Daltons. Another factor is that a molecule needs to be lipid soluble in order to pass through. Essential oil constituents are both small enough (less than 300 Daltons) and lipid soluble. One of the heaviest essential oils, Clary Sage, weighs in at 308 Daltons. The reason they are so light is because of their volatility. During the distillation process only constituents that can be carried up with steam become part of the essential oil distillate.

Cancer is another area that has lots of claims with the use of essential oils but little actual published studies. A study published on August 8, 2013 from the US National Library of Medicine and the National Institutes of Health (www. ncbi.nlm.nih.gov) entitled, "Composition and potential anticancer activities of essential oils obtained from myrrh and frankincense" stated, "...specific components of myrrh and frankincense essential oils are capable of inducing cancer cell apoptosis. For example, sesquiterpenes have anticancer activities that are likely to arrest the proliferation of prostate cancer cells in the G0/G1 phase." Plainly put, they have found that the use of myrrh and frankincense essential oils caused cancer cells to start to die.

While all of this is fascinating, it is important to be your own best advocate. When you understand that essential oils help support cells, it may also interfere with a protocol your doctor has you on. It is imperative to check with your doctor if you are currently on any specific pharmaceutical regimen before you start embarking on any heavy use of essential oils. Essential oils support and regulate healthy bodies. When major sickness is involved you must consider the work ahead. There may be major changes that need to be made in your lifestyle and diet along with your medicinal choices. I will state it again; you are your own best advocate. Be smart, do some research, and then do what is right for you.

Lesson #5
CAN PEOPLE OVERDOSE ON ESSENTIAL OILS?

Is an overdose on essential oils possible? Yes and no. You cannot overdose on most essential oils when used properly, however if used incorrectly you might cause harm to your body. As a more common example, a person may get sick from ingesting, continually over several days, an essential oil that is not for consumption. One common oil that I see people ingesting that should not be ingested daily (only small amounts every now and again are OK) is Tea Tree oil. Even though it has been listed as a GRAS (Generally Recognized as Safe) oil by the FDA it is high in terpenes, which are hard for the kidney and liver to digest. It is fully OK in small quantities but just don't start ingesting 4-10 drops a day, every day. Be smart and read the labels on the bottles. When using certain essential oils topically, you may use too much and have a dermal reaction. See Lesson #6 and #25 for more information.

Lesson #6
CAN PEOPLE BE ALLERGIC TO ESSENTIAL OILS?

I hear all the time, "I can't use Lavender essential oil because I am allergic to all lavender." Can people actually be allergic to the essential oil of a plant? Basically, no. Simply put, pretty much all allergens are from proteins and/or polypeptide nitrogenous molecules, which are typically 100 to 1,000 times larger than essential oil molecules in both size and weight. Also, there have never been any documented cases of an antibody response to the use of an essential oil.

Put simply, allergies occur when an antigen (something from the outside world) enters our bodies and our body over reacts thinking it is dangerous even though it is technically benign like grass or cat dander. If you think about the items humans are commonly allergic to, they really are not dangerous in and of themselves. However, for some reason, a person's immunity will freak out and think it is dangerous and views it as an antigen (a bad thing out to harm us). That antigen will then be attacked by our body's immune system by the formation of antibodies. Those antibodies then bind to the antigen to try to get rid of it. In order for an antibody to bind to an antigen it must be able to form a protein. Essential oils are too small. There are no proteins and nothing for an antibody to bind to.

If a person is new to essential oils, there is zero way he or she is having a histamine reaction unless they were introduced to the plant oil at some other time without knowing it. Because this was all hypothetical, we have to remember that essential oils are too small to have any antibody bind to them in the first place except in the rare case of hapten. The question would then be, "What exactly is a person who claims to have an allergic response to essential oils experiencing?"

There are some studies done on the individual constituents of essential oils, particularly hapten, also know as cinnamaldehyde. This individual constituent is found in Cinnamon Bark and comprises about 90% of the essential oil. Because the individual constituent can then combine with other proteins found in the skin, the immune system will sometimes recognize it as an allergen. The reaction presents as a dermal sensitivity, which technically is not an allergen. If you place any oil that is considered "hot" or "spicy" directly on the skin you risk dermal sensitivity in the form of redness and/or rash. This dermal response may also happen with other essential oils that are considered "hot" oils, such as Oregano and Thyme and may also present in highly detoxifying oils such as Lemon or Grapefruit.

Another way a person may think they are allergic to an essential oil is when the "placebo effect" happens. A person who is very allergic to the lavender plant has trained their sense of smell to alert them to the smell of lavender, should they come in contact with it. Our bodies may have a "ghost" or placebo effect reaction based simply on our mind telling our body we should react. This is known as a Psychosomatic response.

These mental responses are some of the strongest reactions our bodies will have. It is why our limbic system has such a huge pull on our lives and why the power of our minds sometimes will out-rank the power of our physical body. This is a real issue. People get so worked up and freaked out that they actually will react even though scientifically, the way allergens work, they would not react.

A woman came up to my table at a health fair who said the moment she walked in, at the other side of the room from where the essential oil table was that had a cold-water diffuser going, her throat instantly seized up and she had an allergic reaction. Interestingly, she hung out at the essential oil table for quite some time, all the while the diffuser was going right in her face. Rather than get into a debate with her about her obviously incorrect notions, I just smiled and had an internal chuckle at the interesting ways in which our bodies respond since clearly she was perfectly fine at ground zero.

Applying essential oils topically in larger quantities may also present as an allergic response. When a larger amount of essential oil is applied to a larger area of the body by way of neat or less diluted methods, a small percentage of people experience an instant rash or redness. This is something outside the normal range of "heat" experienced in this technique from the use of the more spicy oils such as Oregano or Peppermint. The common reason a dermal rash may occur is due to the amount of chemical toxins currently present in the body or on the skin from using chemical-laden products. The essential oils are doing their job by attacking all the chemicals and the skin gets caught in the crossfire. The rash will subside. However, it is a good indication as to the toxicity of the receiver.

Toxic Release is also considered detoxification, but is based on the essential oil's ability to pull or push toxins out of the cells. As humans we are bombarded daily by petrochemicals and other synthetics in the foods we eat, the air we breathe, the medicines we take, and also the products we use on our skin. These man-made, unnatural chemicals are major endocrine disruptors and may be the cause of the decline of our overall health.

Essential oils (the good guys who are ready to fight) are highly volatile and are naturally inclined to chase down free radicals (the bad guys or toxins). When you place an essential oil on or in your body, they go after these free radicals to murder them off. Your body needs a place to dump these bad guys. Normally your "sweeper" is your kidney and liver. When you first start using essential oils, your body will most likely be overrun with too many bad guys. Your body will then need to look for a back alley to dump the excess bad guys after they have been "offed" by the good guys.

It is at that point that you may experience what is called a vital energy flush. Vital energy is our skin and the feelings associated with our skin such as fever, chills, rashes, headaches, sweating, redness, and lightheadedness, all of which can mimic symptoms of cold, flu, and often allergies. These symptoms are different than what they are mimicking, however, in that they only last a short amount of time. You will experience vital energy detox for a couple hours at most.

The only toxic release symptom that tends to stick around a bit longer when first using essential oils is headaches. Depending on other toxic substances you place in and one your body on a daily basis, this can last 1-2 weeks. The best way to help assist the good guys in getting rid of the bad guys is to drink 80-100 ounces of water per day whenever you know you may experience a toxic release. Adding a drop of Lemon essential oil may also help aid the flushing of toxins, so drink up!

Finally, a person may experience a dermal toxin reaction. This is where the essential oil is reacting to other lotions and toxins already on the skin. Much like the toxic release as noted above, a dermal toxin reaction is based only on the current synthetic chemicals on the dermis layers of the skin. Essential oils will readily go into action to eliminate inorganic matter such as synthetic fragrances and lotions that we liberally apply onto our largest organ, the skin. They are only trying to do their job by bringing organic balance back to the body.

When a person chooses to embark on the use of essential oils it is typically due to their desire to rid their bodies of harmful chemicals. A major first step is to do an inventory of the products they are currently using on their skin and swap them out for chemical (synthetic) free versions. See chapter 8 for Topical Use recipes including face washes and moisturizers, skin balms and serums, perfumes, and other personal care recipes.

It is important to be aware of all potential responses to essential oil use, both in small and large amounts. Know your body and always have a carrier oil present to calm any response that feels uncomfortable. If you use an essential oil and constantly react negatively, you are welcome to discontinue use or try using a smaller amount with a carrier to allow your body to detox more gently. There is no set number of days a detox should begin to subside as everyone is different and we all have a different level of toxicity. You are your own best advocate so do what you feel is best for you. Do not continue using an oil if it makes you uncomfortable beyond normal detox range.

The absolute truth, in a world of non-absolutes, is that our bodies are amazing. They are constantly in a state of homeostasis, which means our body is always trying to regulate back to what it thinks should be normal. Essential oils are constantly trying to obtain this, too. So while we may have an opinion about this and may think one way, we will be presented with clear facts that state otherwise. There is actually a word for this. It is the idea of "prabhava" (pra-VAHV) which means even though something on paper states one thing, when we see it work itself out in life, we know it to have innate characteristics that go against what we think it should do.

A great example of prabhava is Frankincense. The scientific analysis of this oil states it is high in monoterpenes, which would be drying, however everyone uses it in their face serums. We know it is wonderful at skin support to help keep it smooth, but based on the data we should think otherwise. Between two people, prabhava would be considered "chemistry." On paper a couple would be considered the odd couple, but in life they make a magical pair. The concept of prabhava is why our bodies and studying all of it continues to astound me. Keep information in your head but always look for the prabhava of life! Let's be armed with science, grounded in love, and always trust our experience.

Lesson #7
DO ESSENTIAL OILS INTERACT WITH
PRESCRIPTION MEDICATIONS?

There are no known drug interactions with essential oils. David Stewart, PhD, DNM, states, "I researched essential oil/drug interactions thoroughly when I was writing my chemistry book and was unable to find a single citation or publication that indicated any adverse reactions between drugs and essential oils anywhere. If there is a problem between oils and pharmaceuticals, it must not be a serious one since no medical reference I checked referred to the topic. There were some precautions about over-using essential oils by themselves, but I found no publication, by a health care authority who uses both oils and prescription drugs, that mentioned any such problems."

You will undoubtedly see conflicting information online. In one instance there is an abstract by Rhiannon Harris regarding Eucalyptus essential oil stating, "Many oils commonly used for respiratory issues, such as rosemary, eucalyptus, ravintsara and bay laurel are high in 1,8 cineole. Cineole can interfere with metabolism of anaesthesia, and should be avoided (both topically and via inhalation) for at least a week prior to any surgeries to prevent complications." (Harris, Rhiannon. Drug-Essential Oil Interactions: Risks and Reassurances. Presentation to Alliance of International Aromatherapists, 17 Dec. 2008. Denver, CO.)

When cross referenced, you will find a randomized controlled trial with 62 patients before using an injectable anaesthesia called an SNRB (selective nerve root block) and the use of essential oils. It was published in 2014 by the Evidence-Based Complementary and Alternative Medicine, Volume 2014 (2014), Article ID 820126. This study found using Eucalyptus essential oil prior to administering the SNRB significantly diminished anxiety in the patients that would then prove it does not interfere with anesthesia, but would help it.

The issue at hand is to know your body and understand the properties of the oils you are using. For instance, if you are on a blood thinner, then you would want to use Peppermint essential oil with caution, as it is a natural circulatory enhancer. Being on a blood thinner or even taking an aspirin regimen along with the use of Peppermint essential oil may cause lightheadedness.

The question of Grapefruit essential oil comes up often as grapefruit juice may increase the bioavailabililty of some prescription drugs, meaning they will last longer in your system. There is no proof and no cited references stating any "grapefruit juice effect" in the use of Grapefruit essential oils. However, because each person is different, and each situation is different, it is always important to check with your doctor and let him or her know what you are doing for your health before you make any major changes in your health regimen.

Lesson #8
UNDERSTANDING EMFs
(Electromagnetic Frequencies)

As stated on nasa.gov, "When you tune your radio, watch TV, send a text message, or pop popcorn in a microwave oven, you are using electromagnetic energy… Electromagnetic energy travels in waves and spans a broad spectrum from very long radio waves to very short gamma rays." We visibly see frequency at just above 1 quadrillion hertz, which is 10 with 15 zeros. This is what we call visible light. Radio waves are just under microwaves at around 1,000,000,000 or 1 billion hertz. Human bodies radiate heat at around 100 trillion hertz or 100,000,000,000,000. Did you catch that correlation between our cell amount and our frequency heat radiation? We have 100 trillion cells in our bodies.

A hertz (Hz), named after Heinrich Rudolf Hertz, who was the first to prove the existence of electromagnetic waves, is a unit that measures frequency. It is considered one cycle per second, whereas a megahertz (MHz) is one million cycles per second. These frequencies can be found in musical tones, radio waves, computer speeds and electronics. Each periodic table element has a vibrational frequency.

Dr. Royal R. Rife (1888-1971) developed a machine called the Frequency Generator, which is now called the Rife Machine (not FDA approved), to pinpoint specific body frequencies, including healthy body frequencies as well as disease frequencies. "What Dr. Rife claimed is that each microbe has its own resonance frequency. With the Rife technology, he bombarded the microbes with light frequency which matched that of the microbe at an intense level. What he said happened was that the microbes would explode or shrivel up and die." Royal-Rife.com 2005.

With the foundation in place, Bruce Tainio (1944-2009) later invented a machine called the BT3 Frequency Monitoring System. It utilized a sensor that measures bioelectrical frequencies of plant constituents. The BT3 machine is still in production and available to purchase through Coherent Resources, Inc. You can see data from these frequency meters in the following chart, and it will give you a perspective of how frequencies work in our bodies.

Today, you may purchase a biofeedback device such as iTOVi® and Compass Zyto® scanners. While they do not offer any frequency therapy, they do offer biofeedback. They read biomarkers that are out of place based on frequencies. Once the reading is finished, the person will be given products to help regulate and correct those frequencies. Biofeedback comes into play the moment you see the results of your reading. The body will go to work when the brain is told there is a problem.

THE HUMAN BODY & FREQUENCIES

Brain Range	72-90 MHz
Genius Brain	80-82 MHz
Normal Brain	72 MHz
Human Body	62-78 MHz
Human Body from Neck up	72-78 MHz
Human Body from Neck down	60-68 MHz
Thyroid and Parathyroid glands	62-68 MHz
Thymus Gland	65-68 MHz
Heart	67-70 MHz
Lungs	58-65 MHz
Liver	55-60 MHz
Pancreas	60-80 MHz
Stomach	58-65 MHz
Colon	58-63 MHz
Susceptible to Colds and Flu	57-60 MHz
Susceptible to Disease	58 MHz
Susceptible to Candida	55 MHz
Susceptible to Epstein Barr	52 MHz
Susceptible to Cancer	42 MHz
Process of Death Begins	25 MHz

One study done by Dr. Royal Rife and Dr. Robert Becker illustrates the power of frequencies and how our bodies are affected by a change in them. Two young men were measured at a healthy 66 MHz frequency. They both held a cup of coffee. One drank some and one did not. The one that drank it had his frequency drop to 52 MHz in 3 seconds. The one that only held it had his frequency drop to 58 MHz in 3 seconds. Our bodies are very sensitive to our surroundings and the things we place on and in our bodies. We are constantly in a state of homeostasis, where our bodies are trying to regulate our system back to normal range. Essential oils may help aid in that regulation.

There is a misconception regarding the frequencies of oils. Some people believe that the higher the frequency, the better an essential oil is. While true, in some instances, it is not an entirely correct statement. Each system in our bodies responds to different frequencies. Use should be based on which system we are trying to enhance or affect. Bones resonate at a different frequency or vibration than our organs or glands do. Using an array of oils with varying frequencies can help support all body systems. Below is a list of oils and their frequencies. There are hundreds of essential oils, and this list contains just a few to give you an idea of the varied frequency ratings.

ESSENTIAL OILS & FREQUENCIES

Rose	320 MHz
Helichrysum	181 MHz
Frankincense	147 MHz
Ravintsara	134 MHz
Lavender	118 MHz
Myrrh	105 MHz
German Chamomile	105 MHz
Idaho Tansy	105 MHz
Melissa	102 MHz
Juniper	98 MHz
Sandalwood	96 MHz
Angelica	85 MHz
Peppermint	78 MHz
Galbanum	56 MHz
Basil	52 MHz

Lesson #9
INTERESTING FACTS ABOUT OUR BODIES

• The adult human body contains around 100 trillion cells.

• Each cell contains a DNA strand that can store up to 6GB of memory, which makes your body's storage capacity larger than all the computers in the entire world combined.

• The adult human body is made up of around 7 octillion atoms. That is 7,000,000,000,000,000,000,000,000,000.

• There are 10 times the amount of bacteria in the human body as there are cells.

• It is estimated that the human body is made up of 60,000 miles of blood vessels, which if laid end-to-end could wrap around the entire earth almost two and a half times.

• The average human body weight is more than 50% water.

• The human brain is made up of 80% water.

• The average human brain contains 100 billion nerve cells.

• Every 3-4 days your stomach lining replaces itself.

• The average person breathes in and out 20,000 times a day.

• Each day, the kidneys process around 2 quarts of waste in the form of bowel movements, urine, and sweat by using about 200 quarts (50 gallons) of blood to filter it all out.

• Over the average lifespan, a human produces two swimming pools full of saliva.

• A pair of feet have a half a million sweat glands.

• There are 7,200 nerve endings in each foot.

Lesson #10
UNDERSTANDING THE ORAC
(Oxygen Radical Absorption Capacity)

The Oxygen Radical Absorption Capacity (ORAC) is a scale supported by the USDA to measure antioxidant capacities of foods and essential oils. The higher the ORAC value, the more a food or essential oil is able to destroy free radicals in the body and therefore retard the aging process and help prevent disease. A study published in 2005 in the American Journal of Clinical Nutrition by Ilja CW Arts and Peter CH Hollman states, "In addition to their antioxidant properties, polyphenols show several interesting effects in animal models and in vitro systems; they trap and scavenge free radicals, regulate nitric oxide, decrease leukocyte immobilization, induce apoptosis, inhibit cell proliferation and angiogenesis, and exhibit phytoestrogenic activity."

Phenols are a main constituent in essential oils such as Clove and Wintergreen. You can see from the list on the next page that Clove essential oil contains the highest ORAC of any known substance on the earth. Measured in micromole trolox equivaments (TE) per 100 grams, the ORAC values are often listed in other publications as measured in "use per liter," which would add another zero to the end of the numbers. In the following table, the essential oil ORAC values are listed in grams. One of the highest ORAC of a healthy food source is found in wolfberries coming in at 25,300 with blueberries at 2,400, to give you a reference. Raw cacao powder is around 100,000. The following information is from Essential Oils Desk Reference, 3rd Edition, 2006, Life Science Publishing.

FOODS & ORAC

Wolfberries	25,300	Plums	949
Prunes	5,770	Broccoli	890
Blueberries	2,400	Oranges	750
Kale	1,770	Red Grapes	739
Strawberries	1,540	Cherries	670
Spinach	1,260	Eggplant	390
Raspberries	1,220	Carrots	210

ESSENTIAL OILS & ORAC

Clove	1,078,700	Cajeput	37,600
Myrrh	379,800	Peppermint	37,300
Citronella	312,000	Cardamom	36,500
Coriander	298,300	Dill	35,600
Fennel	238,400	Celery Seed	30,300
Clary Sage	221,000	Mandarin	26,500
G. camomile	218,600	Lime	26,200
Cedarwood	169,000	Myrtle	25,400
Rose	160,400	Cypress	24,300
Nutmeg	158,100	Grapefruit	22,600
Marjoram	139,905	Hyssop	20,900
Melissa	134,300	Balsam Fir	20,500
Ylang ylang	130,000	Niaouli	18,600
Palmarosa	127,755	Thyme	15,960
Rosewood	113,200	Oregano	15,300
Manuka	106,200	Sage	14,800
Wintergreen	101,800	Cinnamon bark	10,340
Geranium	101,000	Valerian	6,200
Ginger	99,300	E. globulus	2,410
Bay Laurel	98,900	Orange	1,890
Cumin	82,400	Lemongrass	1,780
Black Pepper	79,700	Helichrysum	1,740
Vetiver	74,300	Ravintsara	890
Petigrain	73,600	Lemon	660
Blue Tansy	68,800	Frankincense	630
Goldenrod	61,900	Spearmint	540
Spikenard	54,800	Lavender	360
Basil	54,000	Rosemary	330
Patchouli	49,400	Juniper	250
White Fir	47,900	R. chamomile	240
Tarragon	37,900	Sandalwood	160

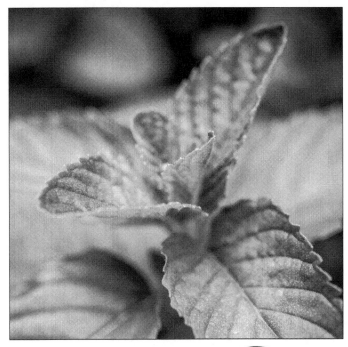

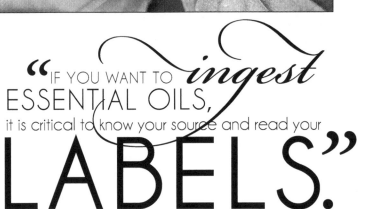

"IF YOU WANT TO *ingest* ESSENTIAL OILS, it is critical to know your source and read your LABELS."

TheEssentialOilTruth.com

*L*esson #11

INGESTING ESSENTIAL OILS

There are several ways to use essential oils internally. Some of the common ways are through suppositories, herbal tinctures, and capsules. Ingesting essential oils via capsule or drinking them in your water is considered controversial topic. Most essential oil users will tell you not to ingest essential oils. They are correct from the standpoint that most essential oils are not meant for consumption. One way to know if an essential oil is truly 100% pure is by checking the label. If it indicates that it is consumable, then you will know it is most likely pure. The label should clearly state that the essential oil can be used as a "dietary supplement" or have "supplemental facts" listed on the back of the label.

With this in mind, you still may have heard that it's not smart to ingest any essential oils. You may have even been told to steer clear of any individual or company that tells you it's OK to ingest essential oils. However, when you understand that the majority of essential oils that are readily available for purchase are adulterated and/or contain toxic chemicals, you can understand why this advice is so prevalent.

The market is flooded with impure essential oils. They are either processed by chemical extraction or they have chemical additives such as synthetic perfumes or alcohol bases as fillers. The majority of essential oils on the market are for the fragrance and general, non-therapeutic aromatherapy industry. You absolutely should not ingest such oils. If you want to ingest essential oils, it is critical to know your source and read your labels.

To check oils you currently use, place a drop on a piece of 100% cotton typing paper. I like to test oils from multiple companies and label each drop above it with the company name. Drip one drop, such as peppermint, from each company onto your paper. Then sit back and watch. If the oil dries super fast and leaves no mark, then it likely has alcohol as a filler. If the oil dries super slow (like 2-4 hours) and leaves a mark, it likely has a non-fragrant oil as a filler, such as Almond oil or Grapeseed oil. If the oil takes a long time to dry and leaves no mark, then most likely, you have a 100% truly pure essential oil.

The problem is that this test is not always conclusive. Unless you are one of the less than 200 trained aromatologists (people who can tell purity through their acute sense of smell), the only way to get reliable, conclusive results is to use an extraordinarily expensive machine to obtain a Certificate of Analysis via gas chromatography. This means that we everyday people are at the mercy of the company selling the oil. Make sure you've researched the company before you ingest the essential oil it provides. The better essential oil companies will provide certificates upon request.

The other issue at play is the simple fact that the naturally occurring chemical constituents within essential oils can be extremely strong. There is a natural assumption that placing essential oils into water for consumption would be a risky thing to do. This is a misconception based on the understanding of how oils work on the surface of our skin. When you get an essential oil on a sensitive area of the skin, such as the face or in the eye, most essential oil users know never to wash away the essential oil by using water, as it will push the essential oils in deeper, causing more heat and pain. We always suggest using rice milk or a carrier oil.

Because of our understanding of how water placed on top of a "hot" essential oil is potentially a bad thing, it is not a stretch to then think placing a drop of peppermint into a glass of water would be a bad thing to do as well. This is not the case at all. The argument will also state that oil separates from the water and will float on top, causing it to be impossible to get the essential oil to infuse into the water. When you drink it, the essential oil could then burn the lining of your throat and stomach.

Skip ahead to lesson #30 on *Essential Oils and Our Circulatory System* to see why this understanding is incorrect (there is an interesting shark fact, too). Yes, a portion of the oils will stay at the top and that is why I recommend gently agitating the glass water bottle before taking a sip. However, if you were to place a single drop of essential oil in a glass of water, wait a few minutes without ever agitating it, and take a tiny sample of water from the bottom of the glass, you would find the essential oil constituents in that sample.

While some of the more "hot" essential oils would not be a great idea to drink, as they could cause a higher sensitivity response, it is something that hundreds of thousands of people do on a daily basis without any issues at all. It is where knowledge of each essential oil comes into play. Consider this: placing one single drop of Cinnamon Bark essential oil into about 32 ounces of rice milk will render some of the tastiest horchata around. Cinnamon Bark is one of the hottest oils, but when used properly can be excitingly delicious! An easier way to consume a drop of Cinnamon Bark without the harsh taste would be to place the drop into a veggie capsule and top off with carrier oil.

Something else to consider is the fact that I said "hundreds of thousands of people" ingest essential oils on a daily basis. This is where the FDA comes into play. You can go onto their website at http://www.fda.gov/ and you will be able to find their statement on GRAS food additives, which stands for Generally Recognized as Safe. If your essential oils are labeled as a dietary supplement, or with a "Supplemental Facts" label, then the FDA has considered them GRAS.

So, think this through: the FDA, who is typically very conservative when it comes to essential oils, is not alarmed at the consumption of essential oils that they have deemed GRAS. The essential oils in question are labeled as consumable under the FDA's specific guidelines. It would then stand to reason that all those "don't-consume-essential-oils-alarmists" out there are just that, alarmists. They have no basis for their standing and it falls apart when you look at decades and decades of thousands upon thousands, if not millions upon millions of people ingesting them with glee and comfort. This again, is based on proper use of each essential oil as directed on the label of each individual type of essential oil.

Bottom line: read the label. If the bottle says the essential oil can be used only aromatically or topically, then do not ingest it. Ever! The best thing you can do is steer clear of any essential oil company that is not providing truly 100% pure essential oil throughout the entire bottle. Below are several of my favorite essential oil-infused water recipes and capsule recipes take from my book *French Aromatherapy: Essential Oil Recipes & Usage Guide*.

Water Recipes:
Create a synergy of essential oils by placing them into a 5mL bottle. After they are blended well, add 1-2 drops of this synergy into a 20 ounce glass or stainless steel water bottle. Gently agitate the water before each sip to ensure proper dispersion. You may purchase a solubol or simply place a Pink Himalayan salt crystal in your water for the essential oil molecules to hold onto. Also try adding the drops to a tablespoon of honey, blend well, and then add the honey to your water. These recipes are for synergies. You would only add 1-2 drops to your water. NOTE: Please only use essential oils labeled for consumption.

The Candy Cane: 10 drops Peppermint, 20 drops each Lemon and Grapefruit

The Creamsicle: 30 drops Tangerine, 5 drops Vanilla

The Fruit Bowl: 10 drops each Lemon, Orange, Tangerine, Lime, and Grapefruit

The Sweet Tea: 10 drops Ocotea, 20 drops Lemon, 40 drops Tangerine

The Zinger: 10 drops Black Pepper, 30 drops Lime

Lesson #12
HEADACHES FROM SMELLS

Are you sensitive to smells? Do you suffer from "scent headaches?" I get an instant headache anytime I am near someone who has on any, and I mean ANY, cologne or perfume. Not fun! I am so sensitive to smells that my close friends and people who work with me know they cannot wear fragrant deodorant, and absolutely no cologne or perfume. Anything from nature though, does not give me headaches.

Take lavender for instance. I can smell the lavender plant all day long, no problem. Give me scented lavender soap or shampoo and I will get a headache. I stay away from all candle shops and I walk super fast on the other side of the mall when I come near those clothing stores that spray cologne on people as they walk in. I am so sensitive that I will know right away if there are synthetic chemicals in any essential oil. I have used 12 different brands and have found only a scant few that I do not get headaches from. That is a big deal to me because it shows me something quite profound about our society and system under which we live.

I understand why many people get nervous about essential oils. They are highly concentrated and super fragrant. So people with sensitivity to smells often think they should not use essential oils. Here's the key: since we know that many essential oils on the market are for the fragrance industry and are cut with synthetic fragrances, which are all created with synthetic chemicals, then of course sensitive people are correct to steer clear of many essential oils on the market.

The average person cannot tell if there are chemicals in a bottle of essential oil. But if you get chemical headaches, then you probably have kept away from essential oils. Know that you don't have to avoid 100% pure essential oils. Only you can know if something is right for you. Pay attention to what your body is telling you. Do your research. Know that all essential oils are not created equal and it is super important to find an essential oil company that you can trust to have integrity and full, throughout-the-bottle purity.

*L*esson #13
OUR RESPONSE TO ESSENTIAL OILS

There are three ways we may respond to the smell of essential oils:

1. You hate it. You say, "Yuck!" when you smell the essential oil.
2. You love it. You fall deeply in love with the essential oil when you smell it or sometimes even just hold it.
3. You have no reaction at all to the essential oil.

What does this mean? Interestingly any major response to an essential oil, either positive or negative, often means your body needs it. We have two major parts to who we are. I like to call it our "hardware" and "software." Our hardware is our physical body. Our software is made up of our emotions, spirituality, thoughts, personality, habits, feelings, and ideas. Our physical being does not care about all the emotional "fluff," it just wants what it wants, when it wants it. This is what Freud called our "id." It is that selfish, primal instinct that drives us.

If you experience a craving and strong desire for an essential oil, almost like your body wants to eat it, then you likely have a physical need for that oil. For instance, people with chronic pain issues will open a bottle of Wintergreen and just love, love, love it. Someone who does not have any pain issues will smell it and may have a neutral feeling about it. Usually the physical will only respond to the needy side, rather than say, "Yuck, I don't like it."

Our emotional side comes from our limbic system. It's our emotional center and is what processes our feelings and thoughts, as well as our long-term memories. It is the storage system for anything good or bad that happens to us. You may smell an essential oil and have a strong, and I mean STRONG, negative reaction to it. Just like your strong positive "id" reaction to loving an essential oil, your strong negative reaction may also mean that you need that essential oil. Strong reactions to, or dislike of a smell likely means that you have some deep-rooted trauma or experience stored up in your body from your life around that smell that you need to work out. This is your limbic system in action.

You may also experience a strong positive reaction to an essential oil, but usually you'll have a pleasant, happy, and loving reaction rather than a strong guttural craving, desire, or intense hatred for an essential oil. This happy reaction means you likely have a wonderful memory of a time in your life where that scent was present. This can all be pretty complicated, but fascinating at the same time. The key is to listen to your body. A strong reaction, either positive or negative, to any essential oil means you need it. Figure out why so you can work toward optimal health.

THE STEAM DISTILLATION PROCESS

A traditional representation of the steam distillation process from 1873. Modern methods are still very similar.

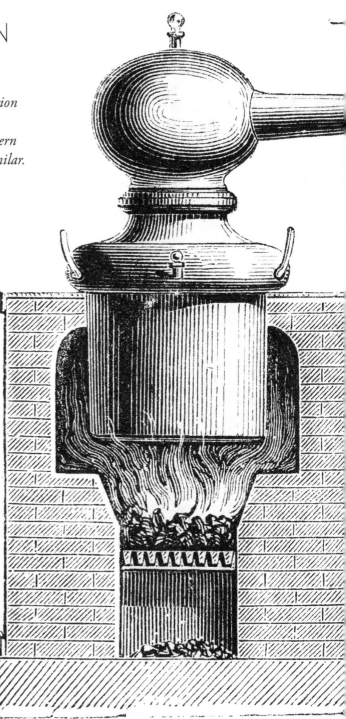

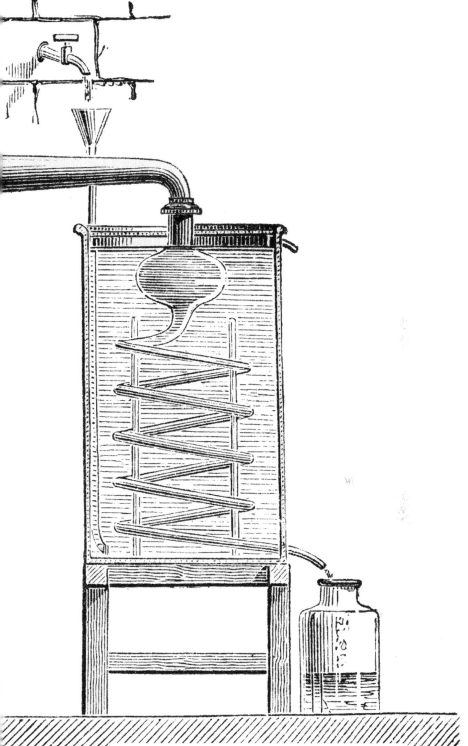

Old schematic illustration of a brass alembic (alchemical still).
Published on L'Eau, by G. Tissandier, Hachette, Paris, 1873.

Lesson #14
ESSENTIAL OIL PURITY

Essential oils are created using several methods of extraction such as steam distillation, solvent extraction, cold press or expression, and CO_2 extraction. The majority of essential oils today are extracted using steam distillation, which we will be discussing in this lesson. There is a lot of misinformation floating around the internet on steam distillation. People may mention various thoughts about first distillation, second distillation, and complete distillation.

Which one is better, how do you define different distillations, and how does it all work? Unfortunately, most information you read is incorrect. Many internet authors do not take the time to research and understand different distillations; they just base their information on assumptions or reiterate ideas from other misinformed posts. I believe that it is critical to know what you are using and if it is right for you. If you are not interested in finding out how your essential oils are processed, then I highly recommend that you either stop using essential oils, or, at the very minimum, read the labels and use them only for aromatic purposes. That's how important it is that you understand production methods.

With all the debate going on about first distills vs. complete distills, it is not really about which one is the right one, or if there even are different distillations, but rather, which complete method, from farming to bottling, does the company practice? The real question should be, was the correct method for that particular plant material used to create the finest quality essential oil to obtain the most desirable end-user action? In other words, does the essential oil work the way you desire it to work?

The reason understanding the distillation process is so important is that many oils from many companies are labeled as pure essential oils. That, however, is a meaningless claim. Federal regulations allow companies to label their essential oils as pure when the product actually contains fillers in addition to pure essential oils. You can't rely on purity claims on the labels. Pretty much every essential oil company on the market states that their essential oil is a variation of the following:

"Pure Therapeutic Grade"
"100% Pure Therapeutic Grade"
"100% Certified Pure Therapeutic Grade"

This is all seemingly fine and well; however, there is no actual certification or regulatory agency in the United States to back up any of these claims. Basically, anyone can call their oils "Certified 100% Pure Therapeutic Grade Essential Oils" or some variation of those words, and no one from the general population would be able to verify if they are what they claim. Now, people are claiming their oils are "Medicinal Grade", as if this grade is even better than "Therapeutic Grade". If a company claims that their essential oils are pure, we would hope that most likely they are, in fact, just that.

If you were trying to sell a product as a high quality product, why would you want to state it as a lower grade? Therapeutic grade implies that there are lower grade essential oils. You will hear people claim this is all nonsense and that there is no such thing as therapeutic grade essential oils. They are either essential oils or they are not. That is not the whole story, though. Just like an egg is not just an egg, nor is water just water. There are different qualities based on many factors. For essential oils there are hundreds of factors that make them what they are.

To say Lavender essential oil is just Lavender would be a mistake. Not only are there many different types of Lavender, there are also different methods of seed selection, farming, harvesting, extracting, and testing methods to ensure the right constituents are contained within the final product. A baking instructor could give 12 students the exact same recipe to bake at home and all would come back with interestingly different outcomes. The same is true with essential oil production. Using the same genus and species of a plant does not guarantee that two different companies will produce the same quality essential oil. Essential oil production is a delicate science that requires a tremendous amount of knowledge and understanding of proper full production from beginning to end.

Even if the essential oils you choose are actually pure, the company does not need to tell you how potent or how exactly they produce their oils. Perhaps the best thing you can do is to call the company to ask some questions, but you need to know more before you can ask intelligent questions. I will be going over a lot of information to help you become more informed in the next few lessons.

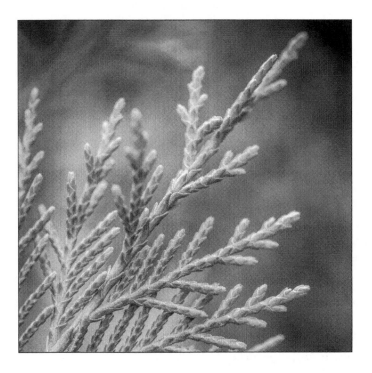

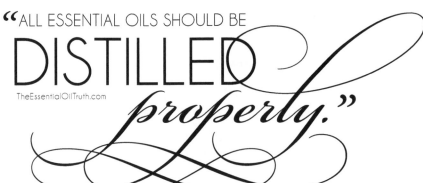

"ALL ESSENTIAL OILS SHOULD BE

DISTILLED

TheEssentialOilTruth.com

properly."

Lesson #15
TRUSTING A LABEL

Consider the simple statistic that France is the leading exporter of Lavender that is labeled "Pure Therapeutic Grade Essential Oil." Sounds simple enough, doesn't it? According to the Lavender Growers Association, there is 100 times more of this oil exported from France each year than is actually grown there! How is that possible? What exactly is in the Lavender essential oil labeled 100% pure? Most likely the bottle contains some amount of 100% pure Lavender essential oil, along with some manmade synthetic lavender perfume as an extender. This is an additive, also known as an adulterant, of the pure essential oil.

Remember, there is no regulation of essential oils. They can call something "Pure Therapeutic Grade Essential Oil" because it contains *some* of it. They are banking on the fact that you will assume that means the *entire* bottle contains only "Pure Therapeutic Grade Essential Oil." In actuality, ethically speaking, they are not lying when they state that it is "Pure Therapeutic Grade Essential Oil" because as long as it contains it, they can state it. It is like listing an ingredient. The marketing trick is that it is done in bold letters so we assume that is *all* that is in the bottle. Unfortunately, often that is not the case.

Lesson #16
HOW THE DISTILLATION PROCESS WORKS

There is a major difference in the types of steam distillations of essential oils. If someone asked you which distill you would want in your oil, the "complete distill" or the "first distill," you will most likely think you want the complete distill. Of course you would want it all, right? Well, that's not exactly true in the essential oil world. Part of the misunderstanding is in the terminology. Technically, in the essential oil industry, all oils would be considered complete distills. This means they are all distilled for the full amount of time that particular single species needs to be distilled. At least, in theory, they should be distilled in the proper manner. For instance, Cypress must go through a minimum distillation time of 24 hours to get all the active constituents into the final product, while Geranium should only be distilled for 1-3 hours. If you define distillation to mean a specific length of time to get the optimal amount of volatile constituents out of a plant material, then yes, you can talk about distillations as a first or highest yield distillation.

Another confused concept is when someone says there is a first distillation, second distillation, third distillation, and complete distillation. People may mistakenly be inclined to think it is the same material being redistilled – something similar to re-using a tea bag. First you create one cup of tea, then take the same bag and try to make another cup of tea, and find that it is way weaker the second time. This analogy is generally incorrect and should not be used when talking about the distillation process. However, sadly, in the world of essential oil production this may sometimes be the case. Doing a second distillation means a plant is distilled first with steam and then redistilled using a chemical pushed through with the steam to extract more of the essential oil. Sometimes, even a third distillation may occur with chemicals. This often happens with Lavandin. This type of extraction is done more that you would think and is a large reason many oils are contaminated with trace synthetic chemicals.

Let us start by defining what the distillation process is without confusing it with the synthetic extraction method. Unfortunately, some companies, who can still label their essential oils as organic or therapeutic grade, try to find shortcuts by raising the temperature or adding pressure to get more essential oil faster. They get more oil to sell, but it drastically alters the therapeutic qualities of the essential oils, also known as the plant's constituents, or molecules. The best companies don't take shortcuts. They use the most costly form of distillation, which is a low-temperature, little to no-pressure, no-solvent extraction method. This method maximizes the therapeutic qualities and keeps the constituents at a level consistent with the finest essential oils, using the standards set forth by the Association French Normalization Organization Regulation (AFNOR) and the International Standards Organization (ISO).

When a plant is grown, if it was grown correctly, it must be harvested at just the right time. You can see more on this in chapters #43 through #48. Once it is harvested, again, depending on the plant, it must either sit for a certain amount of time, or be processed in just the right way; otherwise the whole process will be in vain. Assuming the plant was grown, harvested, and placed correctly into the still, the distillation part is what is in question.

Generally speaking, plant material is distilled for a specific length of time, from 1 hour up to 16-22 hours. The most potent, or what is called the volatile part of the essential oil, that which readily leaps into the air, is extracted during the first part of the distillation process. To understand why the first distill is the most volatile, you need to understand a bit of chemistry, but basically it works as follows: each plant contains thousands of different natural chemical constituents. Some of these constituents contain the best therapeutic qualities, or actions of the essential oil, while others have little to no therapeutic qualities.

They all, however play a roll, and work synergistically together. While one essential oil would need every single constituent, others work better with a higher percentage of a particular, more volatile constituent. Each one of the constituents within the plant material has a different boil rate. The most volatile constituents always boil at a faster rate, meaning they will boil first (during the first part of the distillation). After the first few hours, the essential oil changes in constituents based on what is being extracted from the plant. As more time is added to the distillation, different constituents are extracted and included in the final product. When you get to the final stage of distillation, at the longest point, the final essential oil will smell more fragrant because those constituents (the sweeter part of the plant) boil last. As a bonus, the distillery will get far more out of that plant material than if they only used the first part of the distillation, commonly referred to as the first distill. Most soap and perfume companies will use the complete distill or even a second or third distill, as mentioned earlier by use of chemicals added to the steam, in their final products because it has the most pleasantly mild and sweet smell.

Creating an essential oil with a sweeter, more mild smell will greatly increase sales, simply because of the psychology of smell. When we test an essential oil by smelling it at the local market, we want it to smell nice. Plus, we like the super low, off-the-shelf price tag, too. When a new oil user smells an essential oil that is really earthy or strong smelling, for most of them, their minds tell them not to buy it. This is why most of the essential oils you find readily available are complete, second, or even third distills. This is also why you can pretty much tell right away if your oil is distilled correctly, simply by smelling it. Most really inexpensive oils may still be called pure or 100% essential oil because they are, in fact, just that. Why can they be sold for extraordinarily low prices? They raised the temperature and pressure to make the process faster in order to get a larger batch. It is still pure, but just doesn't contain the constituents we need to better support our body systems. They are great to smell, but they won't do anything for you in terms of real health and well-being.

The litmus test in determining the constituents of a final essential oil batch is in the library of past batches owned by the laboratory testing the oils. Many labs are sorely lacking in their library volumes, so just because a lab states they can test the constituents of an essential oil does not mean they have the means (library) to appropriately read all constituents correctly.

In layman's terms, if you got robbed and you lived in a small town and the only thing you had was a fingerprint from the thief, you'd need to bring it to a police department to find a match. If you went to the small town police department that did not have access to the larger database of national fingerprints, this small town would have a much smaller database based on the people they have already processed for past crimes. They may even have a general fingerprint database from the most notorious people sent in from other cities. The problem is you are most likely out of luck. If your thief does not show up in their database, you won't know who it was. Or worse, you could end up with a wrongly accused person. The better way to find a match would be to go to a large city police department to have your thief fingerprint analyzed.

When an oil is analyzed, basically the markers that it is analyzing is like a fingerprint. It is actually more like multiple fingerprints because there are multiple constituents within a single essential oil. The fingerprint data then needs to be compared to all the other data in the database. Let's say a brand new species of plant life was made into an essential oil and it was sent to a lab for analysis. They might say, "Well it is spiking in this area and showing other spikes in that area but we are not 100% sure." It could then get wrongly accused of being a different constituent. It also has to do with what that lab mostly processes. If it processes mostly petrochemicals, which are usually synthetic plastics as opposed to natural plant chemicals or phytochemicals, they will still try to match them. The machine wants to match whatever it is testing to the data that is already stored in its library. The machine cannot make up things; it's a machine. It has to have a litmus test. It has to have something to match it to. That is what a library is. When you use a library that is smaller, you are going to get potentially inaccurate outcomes.

When you are looking at an essential oil that is found in nature that is widely produced, you will find from each company, based on how they were seeded, cultivated and processed, very different final essential oil molecule levels. If you send it to a lab that does not have a large enough library, you are going to run into some issues. Point being; get to know how your essential oil company processes their oils from farming methods clear through to bottling.

*L*esson #17
THE RIGHT METHOD OF EXTRACTION

Now that we understand how distillation works, which distill is best: a complete distill or first distill? That is not necessarily the question to ask. The better questions are which version is best for *you* and how does the company you use process each specific oil? Assuming the companies you are looking at do not add fillers or use chemicals in any of their processing, the essential oils can be considered pure. The real issue is not necessarily the distillation used, but if the company used the exact right method of extraction for each specific essential oil. The fact is, when speaking about different distillations, they are just different. With each essential oil you try you will need to find the one with the action you desire the most. Some that are not distilled correctly may still work, but may take more drops to work in the way you need them to, or sadly may just smell nice and have zero health effects at all.

Essential oils that are distilled to a weaker action are also milder in smell and milder in effect, so they are great for children when just starting out. On the other hand, you use less of a properly distilled essential oil. One drop will fully infiltrate every single cell with 400,000 molecules in 20 minutes. Did you catch that? Remember, we learned that we have 100 trillion cells in our body, and in 20 minutes one drop that contains 40 million trillion molecules will completely cover your entire cellular makeup, with 400,000 molecules in each and every cell in your body.

I know many people who have tried an essential oil that was distilled to have a greater, more volatile action and it was too strong for them. In a case like this, I just recommend using one drop on the bottom of their feet for the first several days to get their body used to the more powerful essential oil. People who are new to essential oil use may use an oil that was distilled to a milder action and may love them and see results right away. Some milder essential oil users can get away with using their oils their entire life because they are using them infrequently. If, however, they are using them as a therapy and applying them daily, after a few months of using them they will begin to realize the oils are not working as well or as fast anymore.

Realistically, you need to determine your usage and why you would like to use essential oils in the first place. Are they just to make things smell nice and a way to help support the body a few times here and there, or are there more long-term desires and needs to use them in your every day life? The specific action of an essential oil will determine its desired results. I have found that Peppermint is one of the most widely discussed essential oils on this topic. All Peppermint needs to be distilled for the correct amount of time, however the way in which it is grown, harvested, and distilled will give you widely varied results.

One of the ways in which I test essential oils is by using Peppermint from a company I want to try. I rub some diluted Peppermint essential oil on the lymph nodes behind my ears and down my jaw line. Within about 5 minutes I will be able to tell if the essential oil was distilled to my needs. There are very few companies that distill Peppermint properly. It is one of the most popular essential oils, so you might assume there would be some standards or regulations in place. There are not. Bottom line: get to know how your body responds to essential oils and then try several companies side-by-side.

Lesson #18
ESSENTIAL OILS AND DETOX

One of the best ways to detoxify your body is from a cellular level. This is where essential oils come in. For true detox, I only recommend using a correctly distilled essential oil that is pure throughout the bottle. Essential oils are a therapy. Oftentimes, people get essential oils for their health enhancing qualities. If you buy oils and treat them like a one-drop-wonder-quick-fix, you are in for a surprise and major disappointment. You cannot keep them hidden away in your cabinet and once you decide you need them, use them once or twice. It is like using a water bottle to put out a house fire. It just won't work.

When I said essential oils are a therapy I meant it in the way any normal therapy works. When you start a therapy of any kind, you don't go in for one session and are then back to normal. You need to repeat your therapy consistently and with a plan, also known as a regimen. Once you get on a regimen your body will detox and your systems will be better supported, but you need to use them regularly. Also, when you feel the first signs of any drop in wellness you need to ramp up your essential oil use. Better yet, seriously view it as an all out war: using essential oils on your feet, oils in capsules, oils in your diffuser, multiple times per day.

Essential oils are massively detoxifying. If you have a lot of oxidative stress such as bad eating, environmental stress, poor air quality, and a low immune system, then when you first use essential oils you will experience detox symptoms. Even kids will have detox symptoms. Some detox symptoms show up in the form of "flash detox" symptoms. A rash will appear for an hour, or you will be headachy on and off for a day or two, while other times you will actually feel "sick" from detoxing. Sinuses will overreact and you will feel flu-like symptoms.

I recommend drinking at least 2/3 your body weight in ounces of water to help flush your body faster. The normal daily recommendation is half your body weight in ounces (a 150 pound person would take the number 150 and divide it by 2 in order to get 75 ounces), however when you are detoxing, you will want to ramp up your water intake. Using the example above, if you are 150 pounds, drink 100 ounces of water every day for 1-2 weeks when you first start your essential oil regimen.

Your detox days will pass soon enough, but it is a great sign that the essential oils are working. They are like little cellular armies that are working overtime to clear out all the toxic buildup in our bodies. Let the armies do their work and you do your part by eating better, drinking more water, getting proper sleep, and cleaning up your environment.

One of the most common addictions humans struggle with is coffee. The morning ritual is enough to keep people coming back for more, day in and day out. When I talk about even the idea of not drinking coffee anymore to my friends, they look at me with darts, venom, and fire coming out of their eyes. The thought alone makes them shudder. Sadly, our culture has tried to tell us coffee is healthy for us. They say it "ups our metabolism", and "gives us cognitive fitness". I suppose it is the healthier option when you have to drive long distances without an option to sleep. You'd be better off hopped up on coffee than falling asleep at the wheel.

The simple truth is that coffee puts us in a cycle of downward energy depletion that eventually leads us to have to drink just a little more each day. The other issue is that most coffee is laced with synthetic chemicals based on how they are grown and processed. I have friends who have gotten their uterus removed, all in the name of quieting their chronic migraines only to find out that their migraines never went away after surgery. They won't even try giving up their beloved coffee to see if it is the culprit. To detox from coffee I recommend the following regimen. This will only take about 2 weeks to fully detox from caffeine. It is worth it so I encourage you to try.

Coffee Detox Regimen:

1. Take a capsule containing a combination of Ocotea, Peppermint, and Dill oils that may help curb your cravings. Blend equal parts in a 5mL bottle, then drip 3 drops in an empty capsule and top off with a carrier oil. Take 1–2 of these capsules per day.

2. Drink a gallon of water with a total of 6–12 drops of Lemon essential oil per day. For each 20-24 ounce bottle of water, use 1-2 drops of Lemon essential oil.

3. At the times when you normally drink coffee, have a warm cup of herbal tea or hot water with fresh lemon and a bit of honey instead. Try to replace your ritual with something more healthful for your body.

4. Get your lymphatic system moving by walking for a minimum of 30 minutes a day. If you are up for it, I suggest sweating it out through 60 minutes of rigorous cardio. Also, try setting your alarm to go off every hour to prompt you to jog in place for 60 seconds.

5. Find a good quality caffeine replacement that's nutrition based. I personally use a product called Ningxia Red® and Ningxia Nitro® that you can find at www.ningxiared.com—it will help replenish and energize your cells.

6. Get a deep tissue massage once a week during detox. After the massage, take a hot water bath with 4 cups of Epsom salt in the bath. Soak for 20 minutes. Epsom salt helps pull toxins from the body.

7. Take an Epsom salt bath 3 times a week for 2 weeks. Pour 2–4 cups of Epsom salt into a hot bath and soak your entire body for 20 minutes, which will help regulate the minerals in your body and pull toxins out. I also recommend using Dead Sea salt. If you have both, do 2 cups of each per bath.

8. When you feel a craving for coffee, practice deep breathing. Lie down on your back, place your hands on your belly, and take a deep breath to a count of 10, so your lungs fully inflate and your tummy rises. Then breathe out slowly to a count of 20, exhaling as deeply as you can. Try to squeeze all the oxygen out of your lungs. Do this 3–5 times. Get up slowly once you're done, because you may feel light headed.

You can do this! Getting off coffee is hard, but so worth it in the end.

Lesson #19

QUESTIONS TO ASK YOUR ESSENTIAL OIL COMPANY

There are several questions to ask your essential oil company before you start using them or start ingesting them. Please do not ingest any essential oils that are not labeled for consumption. I have spoken to several major brands over the phone that said often times they need to recall items. The reason is, while they can try to audit the farms they buy from, they simply cannot control every factor such as land contamination, what seeds are being used, pesticides, and processing methods. Yes, they can "test" for purity, but often times there are traces of chemicals that they cannot test for or that pass through as pure.

Your goal is to find a company that exceeds regulations. I have friends who literally were getting sick from the oils they were ingesting until I implored them to please stop. It is why you see most articles adamantly stating to never ingest essential oils. It is not because of the essential oil itself, it is because of the potential and real threat of toxic synthetic chemicals even in what are considered "pure" oils. Other companies can claim to be pure, but "pure" is a relative term in the essential oil industry. The best thing to do is call your essential oil company and ask some questions. They will readily answer them, however usually you have to ask for a supervisor or someone who has been with the company for a while.

Questions to Ask an Essential Oil Company:

1. Do they provide complete distill or first distill oils? While this is a hot topic shrouded in confusion, the real question should be: Do they personally distill each oil the way it is supposed to be distilled, for the highest levels of medicinal grade constituents? This is a tough question because no company is going to honestly tell you if they don't distill an essential oil properly. The other questions will help you determine if a given company's oil should be considered in your regimen.

2. Do they distill their oils using solvents? If so, which ones?
Some essential oils, such as Jasmine, must be extracted using chemicals because that is the only way it can be extracted, which would technically be considered an absolute. The only way to know for sure is through your sense of smell and multiple purity tests using a high quality laboratory with an extensive library.

3. Do they distill their own oils or purchase from 3rd parties?

Most companies buy from 3rd parties. Very few companies distill their own. It may be worth your time finding out how testing of the final oil is done. I recommend using a company that uses only the highest standards based on the French standard, not the American, which is very different.

4. Do they bottle their own oils?

Most companies will bottle their own oils, however the oils themselves are purchased pre-distilled and are shipped via large containers. You may want to ask questions 5-11 to find out more about the ways in which your company ensures quality.

5. Do they own their own farms?

There are very few companies that own their own farms. Several companies co-op with farms and some have full control. If they do not own their own farms, what controls do they have in place to ensure quality?

6. Do they provide the seeds to the farmers?

A best practice would be to use seeds from the last year's harvest, choosing only the choicest seeds from the plants that tested at the best constituent levels. Many companies will use hybrids or GMO seeds for higher yields and stronger, more durable plants. This is a very important question to ask.

7. Do they know what pesticides are being used?

All farms should be using essential oils as their pesticides. Most do not know the answer to this because they cannot control the farm they buy from, or the surrounding farms.

8. Do they know if the ground is organic?

Most companies will say it is organic if it has been 4-7 years. It must have been organic for a minimum of 50 years to be considered truly organic. I realize this may seem unrealistic, however, this is the true organic standard. Part of the issue with organic standards is that they are standards. Not above standard. Another thing to consider is a farm can have organic land and practices, yet use non-organic seeds (GMOs or other modified seeds). The product could still be labeled organic, even though the DNA makeup of the plant material is not good.

9. Do they discard any mistakes or are they resold to other companies?
Again, this may also seem unrealistic, but ethically speaking, all mistakes should be either dumped or used as pesticide or cleaning agents around the farms. Sadly, most distilleries sell the oils to the highest bidder, or simply sell them to their customers and wait for enough people to complain and then they recall the batch. I realize business is business, however there are some companies who do not resell sub-par oils.

10. Can you visit the farm to see how the oils are made and take a tour?
The majority of companies do not have access to any farms that they purchase from simply because they are using a broker. There are a few companies that have access to the farms but they would not be open to the public to tour. Very few companies do own their farms and you can readily tour any of them. It is quite a thing to be seen and they will answer any question you have.

11. Are the distillation drums cone-shaped or dome-shaped at the top?
Cone shaped is better, most use dome. Other companies usually do not know this information, so ask if there are any photos of their distilleries on the walls in their corporate headquarters or in any of their marketing materials.

12. Do they test each essential oil batch for purity?
Most will say yes, however, this usually means they got a certificate of analysis from a broker. Find a company that tests every batch of oil for purity and specific constituent levels using above-standard testing. The best standard would be to use either the Central Service Laboratory or the Albert Vielle Laboratory, which are both AFNOR (Association French Normalization Organization Regulation) certified labs and then are fully analyzed by a specially trained chemist on the interpretation of the outcomes.

13. Is testing done in-house only or do they also do 3rd party testing?
Some companies mask their own in-house testing facility with a name other than their company name so it looks like it is a 3rd party. Ask and they will tell you. Find a company that uses true 3rd party testing through a reputable lab, such as the Central Service Laboratory or the Albert Vielle Laboratory.

14. Can they provide you with a Certificate of Analysis?
It is almost impossible to get these from any company because it is proprietary information. General ones are available online and some companies offer a

full range of their certificates from past batches, but these are usually from the brokers and not of their own testing. When you tour some farms and distilleries you can see actual certificates from recent batches.

15. Do they have any trained aromatologists on staff?
There are less than 200 trained "nose" people, who have such sensitive senses of smells that they can tell if there is anything adulterated in an essential oil. Find out if your company has one or more of these people on staff.

16. Do they test their oils side-by-side with oils from other companies?
This is extremely expensive and I know of very few companies that actually do this consistently, if at all. However, it is worth asking.

17. Do they test for when the peak harvest time is?
Oddly, because most companies are not involved in the distillation process, they also do not care about the harvest process. Harvesting time is so important and makes a major difference in the constituents that end up in the final essential oil.

18. Do they ever have to recall their oils?
This happens more than you would think. When a million dollar mistake is made, it is something hard to swallow, so most companies will wait until enough people complain before they recall an item. It is important to go with a company that ensures that bad products don't go to customers in the first place.

19. Do they recommend to NOT ingest their oils?
If they are non-consumable, this may be a giveaway that there are some contaminations or fillers in their oils. Use your best judgment. I have been told by a well known company that even though their oils state clearly, "Not for consumption", they assured me that their members consume them all the time without any issues. No thank you. I highly encourage you to only consume essential oils that are clearly marked as a dietary supplement.

20. How many single, non-blend essential oils do they carry?
A good essential oil company who is truly invested in the industry will carry upward of 80-100 or more essential oils singles.

21. What sustainable practices are in place for their global footprint?
Do they use only sustainable methods of farming and are they conscious of the global impact, in terms of the human and carbon footprint they leave?

*L*esson #20
THE UNDERBELLY OF MARKETING

After understanding the differences in distillation processes, this question always comes up: why would these companies sell weaker essential oils, sometimes at higher prices, than companies selling stronger ones when they know the stronger ones are more volatile and contains higher levels of the healthful constituents? They are all likely well aware, however, processing a stronger distillation is more expensive and takes more fine tuning. From a marketing perspective, when I teach on the subject, I will pass around three to four of the same type of essential oil, such as Peppermint, all from different companies. They all have their labels hidden. Only one, from my experience with the oils, is distilled correctly. I then ask the group three questions:

1. Which essential oil smell do you like better? They always choose the sweeter smelling ones that were distilled much longer or perhaps incorrectly and have sweeter and milder aromas. Based just on smelling alone, everyone will always choose a nicer smelling oil. That is just a fact and is why you can only find these weaker oils in markets. The stronger distills simply won't sell because, based on smelling them, they are really strong and pungent, and usually more earthy smelling.

2. What do you think of when you see a title with the registered trademark symbol after it? The symbols look like this: ® ™
People answer that it looks official somehow. Most do not know exactly what those symbols mean but they do know that it is some sort of seal that states the company did something official to get that mark. The interesting thing about those symbols is that they just mean no one else can use that specific copy, name, or logo.

3. If you could see the bottle, they all say they are therapeutic grade essential oils. What does that mean to you?
Everyone assumes that means they are all standardized somehow and that the entire bottle contains 100% of that essential oil. One of the companies I use in this test does have chemical synthetics. They are all amazed and shocked to find out it is OK for a company to put that label on there even if it is just one of the ingredients but not necessarily the only ingredient.

It has nothing to do with any outside agency officially stating that they are legitimate. I could start a company that states, "Jen the Mind Reader™" with a tagline stating, "Reading the Minds of Celebrities®" and some people

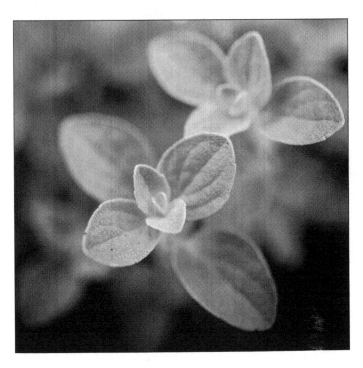

"Get to know your
ESSENTIAL OIL
COMPANY
ON A *deeper*
LEVEL."

TheEssentialOilTruth.com

may be inclined to think it is true, simply because of the little "TM" and the "R" with a circle around it. It may be true too, because once when I was eight years old I guessed correctly several answers prior to the celebrity's answer on a televised game show. Is that ethical? You may decide for yourself; sadly, that is often how companies and their marketing team may justify how they label or promote their products.

There are several other issues at hand when it comes to marketing. Any company that labels their oils as pure therapeutic grade essential oils should be able to state that because all distillations, if done properly, are technically pure. They do not have to prove that they cultivated or harvested the plant material correctly. Even if there are traces of chemicals in them they can still be labeled as pure. The FDA will allow marginal synthetic chemicals in items that are labeled pure. The same is true with labeling something as organic when there are trace chemicals. Trans fat labeling is another slippery slope in the labeling world. A box of cookies can have a huge label on the front that states TRANS FAT FREE, however, when you look at the ingredients on the back of the box you will see listed hydrogenated or partially hydrogenated oils, which are trans fats. How can they do this? Government regulations. It is just how it is.

Companies usually have a goal to produce the best quality. There are three things important aspects in any business and no company can have all three: great quality, great price, and great service. If you want the best quality and great service it will not be at a low price. If you want great quality at a great price, it may take much longer to get or the customer service may be lacking. If you want a great price often the quality and the service are bad. You can't have all three at once in most cases. You have heard it time and time again: you get what you pay for. To think you are getting top quality from a $5 bottle of Frankincense just because it says therapeutic grade on the bottle would be a poor lack of judgment on your part. Look for great quality and great service, at a fair price.

Here is the rub: companies have figured this trick out. It is another marketing strategy. Bump up your prices, slap a quality label on there, and sell a less expensive product. They laugh all the way to the bank simply because the unknowing consumer could not comprehend why anyone would willingly lie to them. We are not wired to think we are gullible or able to be duped. Tell that to the milk industry or the wheat industry. Drink at least 8 ounces of milk a day to keep strong bones, yet the USA has the highest rate of osteoporosis on the planet and we consume the most animal milk on the planet. That is another topic for another book, but I am trying to get you to wise up and think for yourself. So, once again, I encourage you to get to know your essential oil company on a deeper level. Find out what is in your essential oils before you invest heavily in using them.

*L*esson #21
SHOULD I USE A STRONGER OR WEAKER OIL?

What do we do with all this information? Figure out what works for you. Switch brands if you have to, in order to find out which essential oils work best for you and your family. People often ask me why I use the brand that I use and believe me; it was a long process of elimination to find the right one. Quite frankly, I want my oils to work, and I don't want to have to use a lot of it to get it to work. The oils I use are mostly all very strong and volatile essential oils, whereas the majority of the companies out there selling therapeutic grade oils are selling weaker distillations.

You will need to decide for yourself, however, for my family and me I will always stick with the one brand we use. You are more than welcome to reach out to me to find out which brand I use. I do not hide it, as I adore the company and I support them fully. I just wanted this book to stay neutral for you to decide on your own. If you do not even know where to start, please contact me. I am an open book and would be honored to help you figure it all out. If you have a friend who gave you this book who is an oil lady, please talk to them to find out more.

Sadly, all other 12 brands of oils I have tested, just sit in a box, never to be used again. If you are interested to find out if the oil brand you use is on my list I am happy to share with you the information on my tests regarding your brand. I so dislike wasting money and time, so hopefully this information will help you figure out what is best for you. If you want to do your own side-by-side comparisons, here are a few things I do on my own that you may try too.

Test #1 The Freeze Test
Freeze the oils before you open the cap. If they freeze they are low quality. You may also then open the caps once for 60 seconds and then place the cap back on and try freezing them again. The oxygen added to the airspace in the bottle will sometimes create a molecular change in certain oils to cause them now to freeze even if they did not freeze before you opened the cap. On high quality essential oils, this should not happen in a normal freezer on most oils.

Test #2 The Filler Test
Take a piece of cotton rag typing or drawing paper and drip one drop of the same type of oil, like Lavender, from a few different brands. Make sure

they are all of the same listed species, such as *Lavandula angustifolia*. Draw a pencil circle around each drop after the drop has fully infiltrated the paper and label it with the brand name or leave the bottle at the top of each drop. If you use the pencil mark method of labeling, be careful that your pencil mark does not come in contact with the oil drop. Check the paper often. If it dries within the hour and leaves no residual mark, then it is laced with an alcohol as filler. If it takes a while to dry but then leaves a slight stain, then it is laced with carrier oil as filler. If it takes around 4 hours to dry and leaves no residue whatsoever, then it is most likely pure. However, this is not a definitive test on purity, as some chemicals will dry clear too. It is really just a test to find out if there is alcohol or carrier oil used as fillers.

Test #3 The Personal Usage Test
We all have something we love using essential oils for. Find out an area of concern in your body that you would like to support. It may be something simple, like helping support your airways from possible histamine responses. It may be that you want some joint support to help ease symptoms of inflammation. There are thousands of areas that essential oils support, so I want you to find the one that is something your body will feel instantly. I personally need sinus support all the time and there is a simple essential oil synergy that helps support airflow in my sinuses.

Creating a sinus support synergy is one of my litmus tests on any essential oil company I choose to test. I buy their Lavender, Lemon, and Peppermint. I add equal parts into a small 5mL rollerball application bottle and allow them to synergize for about 24 hours. Then, I take the synergy and rub it on my skull behind my ears where there are several lymph nodes, and then a little more just under my earlobe on my neck where there is another lymph node. Within about 30 seconds I can tell the action of the oil and within about 10 minutes I will know if the essential oil company distills their oils in the way I personally need them to work. To date, the 12 companies I have tried have all failed except one. Why? My only explanation is in the way the company distills their oils and controls the entire process.

Whatever brand you decide to use, please call the company to find out as much as you can before you start using their essential oils. You are always welcome to connect with me and ask any questions you have. I have listed my resources and educational groups on the last page of this book. My hope is that you know what you are putting on and in you and your family. Essential oils are serious stuff and should be used with care, caution, and as much education as you can possibly get.

Lesson #22
WHAT SAFETY PRECAUTIONS SHOULD I USE?

There are several safety precautions to be aware of when using essential oils. It is important, first and foremost, to read the label before you use it. Some oils are considered "hot", which means they will feel like they are burning when applied. The most sensitive areas on our bodies are thin-skinned locations, like our faces and genital areas. Essential oils should always be diluted with a carrier oil when applying to a sensitive area. A carrier oil is a non-fragrant oil such as Olive or Grapeseed oil. There are many different types of carrier oils and it is important to find ones that work well for you. Don't just use one.

As an example, Coconut oil is great for the lower dryer parts of your body. Grapeseed oil may be a better option for your face, neck, and chest area, as it has great balancing properties for oily/dry skin. In any event, all carrier oils, even the olive oil you cook with can and should be used when an essential oil gets too "hot." I have a small bottle in every room just in case an essential oil gets in my eye by mistake, or if I get some on a sensitive area on myself or on my child.

If you get an essential oil on a sensitive area, the best way to placate the burning sensation is to apply a carrier oil or rice milk. For instance, if you get an essential oil in your eye, do not flush it with water. You will be forcing the essential oils deeper into your eye, causing the burn to now feel like an inferno. The best thing to do is flush it with a carrier oil or rice milk. We already covered this, but reading the label and knowing how to use each essential oil is an important safety precaution, especially in the area of ingestion. Keep all of your essential oils away from children. Companies who are most reputable will have childproof caps on essential oils such as Wintergreen or Hyssop.

Sun exposure is not recommended after the use of essential oils that are considered photosensitive oils. A general rule-of-thumb is to take caution when using any citrus essential oils. Use sunscreen or do not go into the sun for up to 12-28 hours, depending on your skin type. Safety precautions should also be used when you are currently on a prescription drug regimen. Please consult with your doctor before using essential oils. Pregnancy, baby, children, and pet safety are other areas of concern. Please see the next two lessons for more information.

Lesson #23
PREGNANCY, BABIES & CHILDREN

The use of essential oils on women who are pregnant or nursing, as well as on babies and children should be done with care and caution. Mostly the reason we use caution when pregnant is because the oils will readily transfer to the baby and could cause issues. For babies and children we must remember that their skin is more tender than an adult, so what feels fine "neat" (without a carrier oil) on you may actually feel like a hot iron on them. It is best to always use a carrier oil on children under the age of 12. The best way to use essential oils on children without the use of a carrier oil is on their feet. On children above the age of two you may use essential oils neat on their feet. For babies, always use a carrier oil.

Each essential oil is different, so there is no one specific ratio to use. If the oil is hot for you, then do a 1 to 20 ratio on a child. If it is mild on you then you can try a 1 to 1 ratio. The best way to use essential oils when pregnant, on babies, and children is to proceed with caution. Go "slow and low", as most practitioners like to say. Keep the oils on their feet and use small amounts. A really wonderful way to use very mild versions of essential oils would be to use their hydrosol, which is the water collected from the steam distillation process. While a hydrosol contains very different constituents and heavier water-loving molecules, they make wonderful substitutes while pregnant or on a newborn. They are also an amazing addition to your essential oil regimen even if you are not pregnant. Hydrosols are covered in more detail in the book "French Aromatherapy: Essential Oil Recipes & Usage Guide."

If you are breastfeeding, you will also want to use caution. Unfortunately, when we have our babies we want to get the weight onto them and off of us as fast as possible. Breastfeeding is the best way to accomplish this. However, if you start drinking peppermint water right away, it may change the taste of your breast milk. This may cause your little one not to feed as well or worse, stop breastfeeding altogether. During the breastfeeding years it is also wise to go slow and low on yourself. Don't worry, the time will come when you can go back to your normal essential oil use. For now, concentrate on using oils that can enhance this season of your life, rather than cause issues.

There are lists and lists of essential oils you should stay away from during pregnancy, however they tend to change. I have found these changes are based on assumption. I sometimes see Lavender on a list and wonder if they meant Spanish Lavender, or did they hear some false information about

Lavender being estrogenic or a uterine stimulant and decide it would be best to keep it on the list. Lavender is a wonderful oil to use throughout your pregnancy and for your child. The Lavender hype is just hype based on a study that was done incorrectly and was later recanted. The bad rap Lavender has gotten is still mistakenly talked about, even in the medical community. Had those doctors done a simple 10-minute research session to find out if the gossip were true, they would stop spreading the false information. Doctors are human. Doctors are fallible. We all are. I have researched and studied the most prominent resources on essential oil use and pregnancy from the most well-respected specialists around and have compiled a list of essential oils to avoid during pregnancy.

Essential Oils to Avoid During Pregnancy

Aniseed *(Pimpinella anisum)*
Basil *(Ocimum basilicum)*
Birch *(Betula lenta)*
Blue Cypress *(Callitris intratropica)*
Cassia *(Cinnamomum cassia)*
Camphor *(Cinnamomum camphora)*
Clary Sage *(Salvia sclarea)*
Fennel *(Foeniculum vulgare)*
Ho leaf aka Ravintsara *(Cinnamomum camphora)*
Hyssop *(Hyssopus officinalis)*
Mugwort *(Artemisia vulgaris)*
Myrtle *(Myrtus communis)*
Nutmeg *(Mysristica fragrans)*
Parsley seed or leaf *(Petroselinum sativum)*
Pennyroyal *(Mentha pulegium)*
Sage *(Salvia officinalis)*
Spanish Lavender *(Lavandula stoechas)*
Tansy *(Tanacetum vulgare)*
Tarragon *(Artemisia dracunculus)*
Thuja *(Thuja occidentalis)*
Wintergreen *(Gaultheria procumbens)*
Wormwood *(Artemisia absinthium)*

Avoid the above essential oils along with any blends that contain these essential oils. There are several other essential oils that should be used with caution, but these are the main ones. Please do your research before using any essential oil during your pregnancy, as each trimester presents different usage restrictions.

Lesson #24
ESSENTIAL OILS & PETS

Are essential oils safe for my pets? Generally speaking, yes. However, animals are more sensitive to essential oils and some do not carry enzymes in their liver to process essential oils high in phenols, found in oils such as Clove, and terpenes, found in Tea Tree. Treat animals much like you would a baby. Go low and slow. Pay close attention to their reaction. They will have a more physical and guttural response. Their sense of smell is more sensitive than ours, so a great way to introduce oils to your pets is to wear them on yourself and then approach them to see how they respond. They will let you know right away if they like it or not.

Always use a carrier oil, such as Grapeseed, when placing any essential oils on your animal. Also, always have a carrier oil close at hand, should your pet respond in a negative way so as to dilute the essential oil more. One of the key factors in using any essential oil on pets (and babies for that matter) is that you find a brand that is pure throughout the bottle. There are several brands that claim to be pure; the people who sell them will also fully claim that they are pure throughout, even if they are not. If you take just a few minutes to research it further you will start to find solid evidence that their statements are not true.

Common ways to use essential oils on your pets is to dilute them in a spray bottle with distilled water to spray on their coat or use them with a carrier oil to rub on their paws. Some pet owners have found great success for stress management through the use of a cold water diffuser and 4-6 drops of calming essential oils mixed in with the water. In some instances you may create a synergy and dilute it with 50% carrier oil and place one drop into their mouth by pulling their bottom lip out. Use only milder oils that are labeled as dietary supplements that you personally would be fine placing sublingual. You may also create a capsule using a single drop of your synergy topped off with a minimum of 10 drops carrier oil. Do not use any more for internal use and this method should only be employed when you need a stronger approach for a specific reason.

Please be very careful with essential oils on your pets if you are feeling unsure, however, essential oil use on pets can be a wonderful experience in helping to enhance the health and wellness of your furry family.

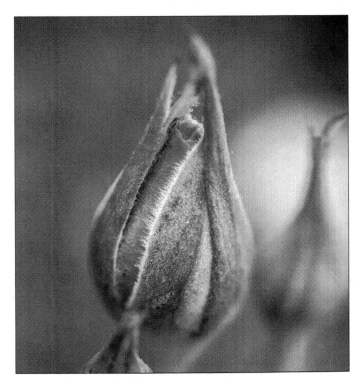

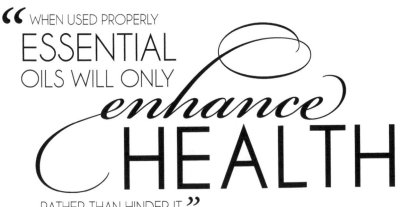

" WHEN USED PROPERLY
ESSENTIAL
OILS WILL ONLY
enhance
HEALTH
RATHER THAN HINDER IT. **"**

*L*esson #25
HAS ANYONE EVER DIED FROM ESSENTIAL OILS?

Over a two-year period, from 2010-2012, there were zero deaths from essential oil use as reported by the NPDS (National Poison Data Systems) as put out by the annual report from the American Association of Poison Control Centers. On the flip side, during 2010 alone there was reported to the CDC (Center for Disease Control) 40,393 drug-induced deaths in just the United States. The CDC also states that 44 people in the United States die every day from overdosing on prescription painkillers. Every day!

JAMA (The Journal of the American Medical Association) did a study from 1993-1998 and found 212,000 deaths in the United States from physician administered procedures as well as properly administered prescription drugs. Essential oils in a negative light are nowhere to be found on the internet database of the CDC, but interestingly they are called-out as potentially toxic by the FDA. Money plays a large roll in our lives and has a lot of power.

The actual deaths from essential oil are incredibly small and, to date, only a scant few have been reported over the last one hundred years. A couple children who somehow were able to ingest 1-2 ounces of an essential oil (eucalyptus was sited on one report and wintergreen on another.) Two adult deaths were reported from women trying to abort their unborn babies. One reportedly drank an entire bottle of Wormwood, and the other Pennyroyal, successfully killing their unborn baby as well as themselves.

As you can see, deaths from essential oil use are extremely rare and the ones that have been reported are from a major lack of common sense. As adults we need to keep essential oils out of reach from small children and we need to educate our older children of their proper use. While essential oils are powerful, when used properly and from a reputable company that only provides the purest oils, they will only enhance your health rather than hinder it.

Lesson #26
UNDERSTANDING PHENOLS

Phenylpropanoids, found in essential oils, are a class of natural chemical compounds, which are a type of phenol. They are varied organic compounds that are combined from the amino acid phenylalanine of plants. They serve as essential components that provide protection and defense, and sometimes provide the color and scent of the plant to help facilitate the pollination process. Phenols are also varied in varieties and have both benefits and detriments to the human body. The phenols found in essential oils such as Clove is called eugenol. There is about 80-90% concentration of eugenol in Clove bud oil and 82-88% in Clove leaf oil. In large doses, 5mL or more at one time, eugenol can be toxic and cause liver damage. The phenol found in Oregano is called carvacrol. The phenol found in Wintergreen is called methyl salicylate. The phenol found in Thyme is called thymol.

What exactly do phenols do for us? They are said to have powerful immunity supporting properties. They are in the essential oils that are considered "hot" oils. Not all essential oils contain phenols. The majority of the essential oils that contain phenols are: Thyme, Eucalyptus, Clove, Cinnamon, Oregano, Bay Leaf, Parsley and Savory. An overuse of essential oils high in phenols may cause dermal sensitivity in the form of rash and redness. Major overuse may cause toxicity. However, when you read about the major dangers of phenols and why it is important to stay away from them, it is referring to man-made phenols, not ones found in nature such as those in properly distilled essential oils.

Lesson #27
UNDERSTANDING TERPENES

Terpenes are found as the primary constituents of many essential oils. They are responsible for the strong smell you find in essential oils like Tea Tree and Frankincense. There are ten different types of terpenes and within each type there are thousands, and sometimes tens of thousands of different varieties. The two major terpenes found in essential oils are monoterpenes and sesquiterpenes. There are also diterpenes and triterpenes found in essential oils, but in smaller amounts, so we will focus on the two major terpenes.

Several monoterpenes have cleansing properties. They are also key in regulating enzymes and act as solvents to dissolve gallstones as well as black grime on our cars and ovens. It is why you can put one drop of lemon onto sticker residue and it will dissolve it in seconds. Monoterpenes are found in the essential oils of Frankincense, Lemon, Grapefruit, Caraway, Orange, Dill, Bergamot, Spearmint, and Peppermint.

Sesquiterpenes act as defense agents as well as contain pheromone-like properties. They also have properties that are cleansing, help support inflammation, and act as calming agents as in the use of pheromones. They are touted by the US National Library of Medicine and the National Institutes of Health as "a class of naturally occurring molecules that have demonstrated therapeutic potential in decreasing the progression of cancer." Sesquiterpenes are the main constituents of Vetiver, Cedarwood, Patchouli, Sandalwood, Ginger, and Myrrh. Sesquiterpenes are also found in lower percentages in Black Pepper and Frankincense along with several other essential oils.

Lesson #28
ESSENTIAL OILS VS. TRADITIONAL MEDICATIONS

When medications are made, they are created mostly as beta-blockers. Beta-blockers enter our system and block our body from "feeling" a symptom. They do not get to the root cause of the symptom; they just help us feel better even when we are not. This can be a somewhat precarious position to be in, because it then confuses and tricks our body into thinking the problem is solved and may lessen our body's ability to heal faster, if at all.

Essential oils work very differently than traditional medications. They have the ability to enter the cell wall because their molecules are so tiny, where traditional pharmaceuticals do not have that ability. A virus can live inside the cell, while bacteria lives on the outside of the cell. It is why you will hear that you can never fully kill herpes from our bodies. You will be able to treat the symptoms and may help alleviate them, but not eliminate them. You will, in time, get another flair-up. It is because it is a virus that lives inside the cell.

Our cells allow essential oils to enter because they are from nature, are so small, and are lipid-soluble. The oils have one goal: to support and regulate healthy body function. It is a good thing that synthetic drugs cannot enter the cell wall. We would be in big trouble if they could, as they would not only kill the bad things, but the good as well. It is the age-old problem pharmaceutical companies face.

Lesson #29
ESSENTIAL OILS & THE BODY SYSTEMS

Essential oils, in the plant form, help the plant often in the same way essential oils help our systems. If a constituent helps regulate, stabilize, or keep predators away in the plant, it often does the same in human cells as well. The following 12 lessons will simply describe a specific system so you are better prepared to understand how your body works in conjunction with essential oils. You will see many oils work well for multiple systems, and many systems are interconnected.

In each chapter you will see a list of essential oils that support the healthful function of each system, and how and where to apply them for the most effective results. For the specific properties of each essential oil and more specific areas they support, please refer to the reference guide from the company you buy your oils from. The lists of essential oils in the following chapters are not meant to be definitive or exhaustive, as each person responds to essential oils differently. You may use these essential oils aromatically, topically, and in some cases internally. Please refer to the product label for proper use of each individual essential oil.

Lesson #30
ESSENTIAL OILS & THE CIRCULATORY SYSTEM

The circulatory system is also called the cardiovascular system. It is our blood transportation system. Blood gives the cells nutrients, oxygen, carbon dioxide, and hormones. These all work together to stabilize the body's temperature and pH balance (called homeostasis) as well as help fight disease. The circulatory system includes the heart, blood vessels, and blood. Because we are comprised of about 7% blood, which circulates throughout the entire body, it is important to support a healthy circulatory system.

Essential oils are, in essence, the blood of the plant. When we consider what our blood is, we will start to realize healthy blood is of the utmost importance. We have a symbiotic relationship with greenery on our planet. We rely on it for oxygen, and it relies on us for carbon dioxide. If the entire human race along with every oxygen-breathing life form perished, all the vegetation on the earth would soon perish, too. If all the vegetation on the earth including algae in the ocean died today, it is estimated that the entire population would perish in less than three days. We need each other. Plant life has something within its cells that we also need. It is not as critical as oxygen, however it can support a more healthful and beneficial quality of life when we start to see the benefits of the plant's "blood" also known as its circulatory system.

How and why does a plant's circulatory system relate to our circulatory system? The essential oils of a plant work in the same way our blood does. It moves within the plant via veins to get critical and functional care to all parts of the plant. It is why you can place a drop of essential oil into a glass of water without agitating it, and the oil will still permeate the entirety of the water within just a few minutes. It is also why when a person bleeds in the ocean a shark can pick up the scent of blood miles away. National Geographic states, "Great whites can detect one drop of blood in 25 gal (100 L) of water and can sense even tiny amounts of blood in the water up to 3 mi (5 km) away."

Essential oils travel swiftly through the plant just as our blood travels swiftly through our veins and arteries. One drop of essential oil placed on the bottom of your feet will infiltrate your entire body within 20 minutes. Just like the essential oil of a plant needs to get efficiently and effectively to a specific location in the plant to support its many functions, so must our blood in our bodies. If we do not have proper circulation, many of our systems and functions will begin to fail or become sub-par in performance, which can lead to sickness and disease.

Using essential oils to support proper circulation is the starting point for all other systems. Support your circulation, and you will be supporting the root of most other functions and systems in your body. Your roots determine your fruits. In the case of your body systems, your circulatory system is your roots.

Essential oils that may help support the circulatory system:
Cassia, Cinnamon Bark, Clove, Cypress, Eucalyptus, Grapefruit, Helichrysum, Hyssop, Lavender, Lemon, Lemongrass, Marjoram, Peppermint, Rosemary, Spearmint, Wintergreen, Ylang ylang

Because your circulatory system runs throughout your entire body, you can effectively access it through multiple methods. Most notable are the areas like your wrists and neck where perfume is applied since there are veins close to the surface and the skin in those locations is thinner. Another effective way would be to ingest the essential oils via capsule or in a beverage on a daily basis to support this system. Please refer to individual oil labels for proper use.

Lesson #31
ESSENTIAL OILS & THE DIGESTIVE SYSTEM

The digestive system starts in the mouth with the teeth and saliva. The entire process is based on breaking down our food into smaller and smaller particles so it may be properly absorbed into the body. In order to have a healthy digestive system there are two important things: the liquid component comprised of saliva, gastric juice, and mucus along with the functional component comprised of the mouth, teeth, jaw muscles, esophagus, stomach, gastrointestinal tract, small intestine, large intestine, colon, rectum, and anus with their various muscular components.

Essential oils can help support all areas of the digestive system and it is important to note that, because our systems are interconnected, we can easily support one system through use of another. For example, if you have unwanted bacteria causing an upset stomach, you can rub specific oils on your jaw line where there are several lymph nodes between thin skin and hard bone. Getting the essential oils into the lymphatic system quickly may help ease uncomfortable stomach issues.

Essential oils that may help support the digestive system:
Black Pepper, Caraway, Cinnamon Bark, Clary Sage, Copaiba, Fennel, Ginger, Grapefruit, Lavender, Lemon, Lemongrass, Marjoram, Nutmeg, Orange, Patchouli, Peppermint, Rosemary, Sage, Spearmint, Tangerine, Thyme

Many essential oils used for digestive system support are used topically as well as internally when the label states the oil is ingestible. For topical use, you may place the oil on location nearest to the area of interest. It may also be applied to the vita flex points on the feet relating to the area, or through application on an interconnected system such as the lymphatic or circulatory system. The lymphatic system can be accessed through our lymph nodes by placing oils directly on the skin where a node is. The circulatory system can be accessed through our feet vita flex points as well as under our tongue. A single drop directly under the tongue will help get the essential oil into the circulatory system and, therefore, into the digestive system.

*L*esson #32
ESSENTIAL OILS & THE ENDOCRINE SYSTEM
(hormones and enzymes)

The endocrine system is directly related to the circulatory system and consists of the glands in the body that secrete hormones and enzymes. Some of the major glands in the endocrine system are the adrenal glands, hypothalamus, pancreas, parathyroid gland, pineal gland, pituitary gland, thyroid gland, ovaries and testes, which is also part of the reproductive system.

Essential oil use can greatly enhance the health of the endocrine system. Because essential oils help regulate the hormones in our bodies, they may mimic the needed hormone in some cases, but in most cases will stimulate a specific gland to regulate the hormones we are in need of. Hormonal imbalance is widespread, and the use of essential oils can help regulate and normalize our system.

Starting in the head there are three glands: the pineal, hypothalamus, and pituitary. Moving down the body, there is the thyroid, adrenal, pancreas, ovaries, and testes. Below is a description of each, along with essential oils that may help support the proper function of that gland.

The **pineal** gland is responsible for the release of melatonin, which helps regulate sleep patterns.

Essential oils that may help support the pineal:
Frankincense, Sandalwood, Cedarwood, Spruce
How to use: Smell the oils, place them in your mouth, on the roof of your mouth, under your tongue, between your eyebrows, on your crown, and/or on the nape of your neck.

The **hypothalamus** is part of the brain, which links the endocrine system to the nervous system by way of the pituitary gland. The hypothalamus regulates hunger, thirst, body temperature, along with sleep and alertness.

Essential oils that may help support the hypothalamus:
Peppermint, Lavender, Cedarwood, Dill, Frankincense, Sandalwood, Marjoram
How to use: Smell the oils, place them in your mouth and rub them on the base of your neck.

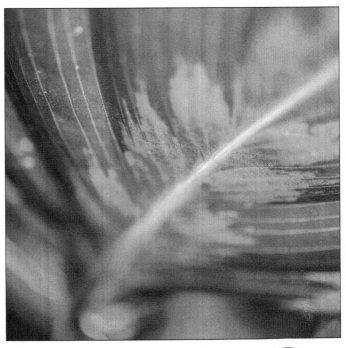

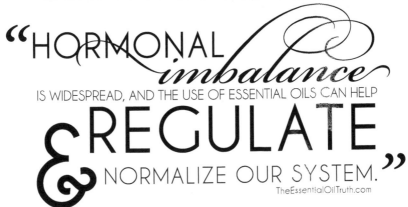

"HORMONAL *imbalance* IS WIDESPREAD, AND THE USE OF ESSENTIAL OILS CAN HELP & REGULATE NORMALIZE OUR SYSTEM."

The **pituitary** gland sits just at the base of the brain and is responsible for regulating growth, metabolism, and reproduction, as well as stress and blood pressure. It also regulates temperature and pain relief. At just about the size of the tip of your pinky finger or a small green pea, weighing in at only 0.5 grams, the pituitary has a big job for such a small gland.

Essential oils that may help support the pituitary:
Frankincense, Cinnamon Bark, Cedarwood
How to use: Smelling the oils is the most direct method. Another great way is to place a drop into your hand and dip your thumb into it and place it on the roof of your mouth for 15-30 seconds. You can also drip a drop under your tongue, apply some in between your eyebrows, on the crown of your head, the back of your head, and base of the neck.

The **thyroid** gland is in the neck and are two lobes connected to each other. The thyroid regulates energy in our body. It also helps our body know how to react to other hormones as they are released. There are four thyroid disorders, with the two main ones being hyperthyroidism and hypothyroidism.

"Hyper" refers to an overactive thyroid and "hypo" refers to a thyroid that produces less than normal hormones. Common symptoms of people with hyperthyroidism are increased appetite, increased heart rate, weight loss, fatigue, diarrhea, heat intolerance, and sweating, along with several other symptoms. Common symptoms of hypothyroidism include weight gain, fatigue, slow heart rate, hair loss, and cold intolerance.

Essential oils that may help support the thyroid:
Geranium, Carrot Seed, Cypress, Myrrh

Hyperthyroid: Wintergreen, Sandalwood, Frankincense, Black Spruce, Lemongrass
Hypothyroid: Spearmint, Myrrh, Peppermint, Frankincense, Clove, Cedarwood, Ledum, Myrtle

How to use: Apply on the vita flex points on your feet at the base of your big toe from your middle toe out to your big toe joint at the widest part of your inner foot. Inhale and in some cases you may ingest, however please refer to the labels.

The **adrenal** glands are located at the top of our kidneys. We have two, and each consist of multiple layers, which produce several hormones. These hormones regulate blood pressure electrolytes, immunity suppression, and sexual hormones. One of the main hormones secreted is called cortisol. It helps regulate metabolism, stress, immunity, and inflammation. Aldosterone regulates blood pressure and volume, along with potassium and sodium levels. Other hormones from the adrenal glands are androgen, noradrenaline and adrenaline.

Essential oils that may help support the adrenal are:
Lavender, Rosemary, Ylang ylang, Bergamot
How to use: Massage on kidney vita flex points on hands (middle of both thumb pad muscles) and feet (middle of both feet). Inhale and in some cases you may ingest, however please refer to individual oil labels for usage.

The **pancreas** is part of the endocrine and digestive systems. It is located just behind the stomach, and produces hormones such as insulin and glucagon, along with a couple other regulatory hormones. Insulin regulates our metabolism of fats and carbs so the glucose from the blood can be absorbed properly. Insulin lowers the levels of glucose in the bloodstream. The pancreas also produces glucagon, which helps elevate glucose in the bloodstream.

Essential oils that may help support the pancreas:
Marjoram, Lemon, Basil, Vetiver, Cypress
How to use: Massage over the abdomen and apply to vita flex points on feet and hands (middle of the palm directly below pinky finger on left hand and middle of foot toward the outside on the left foot). Inhale, and in some cases you may ingest, however please refer to individual oil labels for usage.

The **ovaries** in the female are below the stomach on either side, near the hipbones. They are responsible for providing the eggs, and they secrete estrogen, testosterone, and progesterone.

Essential oils that may help support the ovaries:
Frankincense, Cypress, Geranium
How to use: For women, create a retention tampon by adding 1-2 drops essential oil to 1Tbs. carrier oil inserted into the vaginal canal nightly for 4 nights. May be rubbed on ankle bones and over ovary locations.

Estrogen and Testosterone Support: Clary Sage
How to use: rub the essential oil on vita flex points over ankles or directly over ovaries for women.

Testes (plural for testicle or testis) are part of the male reproductive system. They are responsible for the production of sperm, as well as the hormone testosterone.

Essential oils that may help support the testes:
Patchouli, Ylang ylang, Spruce, Copaiba
How to use: rub essential oils diluted with a carrier oil directly on the testicles and use aromatically.

Estrogen and Testosterone Support for Men: Clary Sage
How to use: rub on vita flex points over ankles or directly on testes with a carrier oil.

Lesson #33
ESSENTIAL OILS & THE IMMUNE SYSTEM

The immune system protects the body against disease and sickness. It detects pathogens and determines the difference between the bad and good organisms. When the immune system is lowered, or underactive, it can result in sickness. A hyperactive immune system will cause the body to start attacking our normal tissue, thinking it is diseased. Inflammation is usually the immune system's first response to infection.

There are several outside factors that may lower the immune system and therefore lower its ability to fight off disease and infections. Among them are sleep deprivation, sugar, ingestion of chemicals such as preservatives and man made processed food additives, improper diet and lack of fatty acids, stress, obesity, alcohol, cigarettes, caffeine, prescription drugs, lack of exercise, too much sun exposure, as well as not drinking enough water.

Essential oils that may help support the immune system:
Cinnamon Bark, Cistus, Clove, Cumin, Eucalyptus, Frankincense, Hyssop, Lavender, Ledum, Lemon, Melaleuca, Oregano, Ravintsara, Rosemary, Thyme

Simply inhaling essential oils will help support our immune system. Applying them topically and internally in some cases are often the more aggressive route when needing to regulate and support proper immune function. The best way is to embark on a daily regimen of essential oil use. Take several oils to make a synergy and create a rollerball and roll on the bottom of your feet and nape of your neck every day.

When you find yourself with a compromised immunity, you will want to support it from multiple angles. Eat well, as in no sugar or processed foods, drink lots of water, and get more rest. We all know these things. Adding essential oils in a more deliberate way may help lessen the time you are down. Consider not only using oils topically on your feet, wrists, and neck, but also use a cold-water diffuser with an immunity supporting synergy. To support it even more aggressively, you may want to create an immunity capsule with 2 drops of a synergy of 3 or 5 of the above oils topped off with a carrier oil, only if they are labeled for consumption, and take 1-2 times a day.

Lesson #34
ESSENTIAL OILS & THE INTEGUMENTARY SYSTEM
(skin, hair, and nails)

The integumentary system is the largest organ in the body comprising the skin, hair, and nails. It amounts to 12-15% of the total body weight. Its function is to protect the body on many levels both internally and externally, as well as to excrete waste through perspiration and create vitamin D from ultra-violet light exposure. It acts as a receptor for the somatosensory system, which is the sense of touch including pressure, temperature, pain, and pleasure.

There are many ways in which essential oils can support the proper healthful function of the integumentary system. For the nails and hair, essential oils have the ability to support the strength and growth. Nail beds can be strengthened by using Lemon, while hair may be strengthened by using Lavender and Cedarwood. Many women love using a few drops of Cedarwood directly on their scalp between washings to keep it smelling fresh.

The skin, being the largest part of our integumentary system, can be supported by many different essential oils. Based on historical fact, the use of Frankincense and Myrrh were the common embalming oils used by the Egyptians due to their ability to preserve skin. It is no wonder that women today use these essential oils as part of their daily face regimen. Lavender has skin soothing properties while Tea Tree has revitalizing properties. Patchouli, Rosewood, and Cypress help promote skin firming while Sandalwood, Helichrysum, and Frankincense support healthful regeneration.

Essential oils that may help support the integumentary system:

Skin: Frankincense, Myrrh, Tea Tree, Lavender, Cedarwood, Peppermint, Patchouli, Cypress, Helichrysum, Sandalwood, Roman Chamomile, Geranium, Jasmine, Ledum, Lemon, Marjoram, Palmarosa, Rosemary, Rosewood, Sage, Vetiver, Ylang ylang

Hair: Cedarwood, Rosemary, Cypress, Lavender, Thyme, Tamanu, Tea Tree, Patchouli, Sage, Valerian, Basil, Geranium, Sandalwood, Peppermint

Nails: Lemon, Tea Tree, Frankincense, Myrrh, Eucalyptus, Grapefruit, Lavender, Lime, Oregano, Patchouli, Peppermint, Rosemary, Thyme

Lesson #35
ESSENTIAL OILS & THE LIMBIC SYSTEM
(emotions)

The limbic system, found on either side of the thalamus directly under the brain, right in the middle of the head, is responsible for several functions our personhood goes through. Why I say "personhood" is because it is not directly related to our hardware (our physical body) as much as our software (our emotional, thought part of our humanity.) While it is responsible for the epinephrine flow (adrenaline), which is physical, the main function is to support the emotions, memories (long-term and spatial memory), motivation, behavior, learning, and the actual sense of smell, which is called olfaction, or the olfactory system.

Essential oils can support our limbic system through aromatherapy by pulling the oils directly into our nose. By deeply smelling them or placing them on the roof of our mouth we can help support such areas as learning, behavior, and motivation. The use of certain essential oils can also help us with our long-term memories and more specifically our emotional response to the world around us. There is much to learn about our limbic system and its limitless ability to store emotional trauma. The use of essential oils can help release that trauma.

Connie and Alan Higley state in the "Reference Guide for Essential Oils", "High levels of sesquiterpenes, found in the essential oils of frankincense and sandalwood, help increase the amount of oxygen in the limbic system of the brain, particularly around the pineal and pituitary glands. This leads to increase in secretions of antibodies, endorphins, and neurotransmitters. Also present in the limbic system of the brain is a gland called the amygdala. In 1989, it was discovered that the amygdala plays a major role in the storing and releasing of emotional trauma. The only way to stimulate this gland is with fragrance or the sense of smell. Therefore, with aromatherapy and essential oils we are now able to release emotional trauma."

Our emotions are a tricky thing. We often feel like we live and die by them. At times, our emotions, can make life insanely wonderful and impossibly unbearable. They can feel out of control, like they somehow control us, yet at the same time we know, deep in our logical mind, that we have the ability to choose our emotional response. The interesting thing however, with all the self-help books and motivational speakers telling us our emotions are a choice is that we all know that is not exactly true. Sure, we can choose to change our mind about how we feel but our instinctual, guttural reaction, when it comes to our emotional response to things, is very real and very knee-jerk.

We live in a world that relies on our five senses: touch, taste, hearing, sight, and smell. The first four listed go through our logical center of our brain first and then our emotional. Basically, when you see a baby, your brain instantly and simply thinks "baby." You might even logically think, "Where is his mom" or "Why is he wearing pink when he looks like a boy?" After these logical responses, usually a split second later, the visual of the baby will go through your emotional center to tell you if you are happy, annoyed, fearful, angry, or any other number of emotional responses. It all depends on how you feel about babies. Logical first, emotional second.

However, let's say you smelled a bottle of baby powder. Your mind will instantly go to an emotional response first. Your limbic system, which is connected to your sense of smell, is the only sense that works in the other direction from every other sense. Our emotions are called on first, and then logical. Armed with this simple understanding we may be able to help promote a more healthful emotional state simply through the use of aromatherapy. Below is a list of oils that may support and encourage you on your path to emotional well being.

Essential oils that may help support the limbic system:

Specific Areas:

Anger: Lavender, Bergamot, Cedarwood, Cypress, Rose, Melissa, Orange, Frankincense, Geranium, Helichrysum, Lemon, Mandarin, Sandalwood

Fear: Bergamot, Clary Sage, Cypress, Fir, Germanium, Juniper, Marjoram, Myrrh, Orange, Roman Chamomile, Rose, Sandalwood, Spruce, Ylang ylang

Sadness: Helichrysum, Geranium, Orange

Addictions: Dill, Peppermint, Black Pepper, Grapefruit, Cumin, Lavender, Marjoram, Nutmeg, Sandalwood

Agitation: Lavender, Ylang ylang, Orange, Rose, Melissa, Cedarwood, Bergamot, Jasmine, Frankincense

Long Term Memory: Rosemary, Basil, Clary Sage, Ginger, Grapefruit, Lemon, Roman Chamomile, Thyme

Motivation: Myrrh, Lavender, Lemon, Orange, Peppermint, Roman Chamomile, Spruce, Ylang ylang

Learning & Focus: Lavender, Vetiver, Ledum, Ylang ylang, Cedarwood, Frankincense, Sandalwood, Spruce

This list is not meant to be definitive or exhaustive as each person responds to essential oils differently. To use essential oils to support our limbic system, it is best to inhale them deeply or simply put a drop on your wrists or bottom of your feet. For aromatic use, try putting 3-4 drops of several different essential oils into a diffuser and sit nearby to enjoy the benefits. A quick method is to drop one drop into your non-dominant hand and with your dominant hand, press your palms together and rotate 180 degrees. Then cup your hands tightly over your nose area and breathe in as deeply and as smoothly as you can three full times. Then rub the leftover essential oils on your shoulders and on the back of your neck at the base of your skull.

*L*esson #36
ESSENTIAL OILS & THE LYMPHATIC SYSTEM
(circulatory cleaning)

The lymphatic system is a part of the circulatory system. It is a large network of vessels that carry lymph toward the heart. It is also an integral part of the immune system and is responsible for cleaning the body of toxins. We have more lymph in our system than we do blood. The cardiovascular system is a closed system with a central pump: the heart. The lymphatic system is not a closed system and has no central pump, therefore is often slow and intermittent. It is why we often will get what is called a "sluggish lymph." This means we are not getting enough activity to stimulate our lymph and will get tired or lethargic. This does not mean that if you sit for too long your lymph will not move at all. The lymph moves based on several factors: any form of general muscle movement, and involuntary movement of the surrounding valves and arteries.

Lymphatic movement is important because it determines how well the immune system and waste system work. Its job is also to transport and absorb fats from the digestive system, as well as transport white blood cells to the bones from the lymph nodes. I like to call my lymph my internal army. The lymph (which is a milky white substance) goes to work for me and I want it to be stimulated. The lymph cleans out the bacteria and flushes out the toxins from my body. Using essential oils to help support a healthy lymphatic system is important because if my lymph grinds to a slow crawl, so do I, in every sense of the phrase. Below is a list of important essential oils to add to your daily arsenal to support a happy and healthy lymphatic system.

Essential oils that may help support the lymphatic system:
Cypress, Frankincense, Grapefruit, Helichrysum, Lavender, Ledum, Lemon, Lemongrass, Lime, Myrtle, Oregano, Peppermint, Rosemary, Sage, Sandalwood, Spearmint, Tangerine, Thyme

Essential oils should be applied directly to lymph node areas as well as ingested only when the label states for consumption. When applying them on a lymph node area you may use the oils "neat" or diluted with a carrier oil. One of the most effective ways to easily access our lymph is to place a few drops of an essential oil on our fingers and rub them on your skull behind your ears and then pull your fingers down along the ridge of your jaw line.

You have some posterior auricular nodes behind your ears on your skull, one at the upper part of your jaw just below your ear called the tonsillar, and several submandibular nodes down your jaw line to your chin. The reason these nodes are easily accessible is because they are between thinner skin and bone (jaw or skull). You can easily create a lymph support rollerball and use it as needed. My favorite lymphatic support recipe is as follows:

Get a 5mL rollerball bottle with a metal roller fitment. Create a synergy using 10 drops each of Lemon, Lavender, and Peppermint, then add 5 drops each of Ledum and Lime. Let synergize for 24 hours then top off with carrier oil. Use this along your jaw line and on your skull behind your ear.

As mentioned earlier in this book, often times someone gets an upset stomach from bacteria and it is far more effective to support it through application of an essential oil on the jaw line lymph than actually rubbing it on your stomach area. This is why learning your systems and how they function can make all the difference with deciding how to use an essential oil and which one to use.

Lesson #37
ESSENTIAL OILS & THE NERVOUS SYSTEM

The nervous system is responsible for controlling the voluntary and involuntary movements and actions, both externally and internally. There are two parts to the nervous system; the central nervous system, which is comprised of the brain, the thalamus as the connector hub, and spinal cord, and the peripheral nervous system, which is comprised mainly of nerves and connects the central nervous system to the whole body. Within the nervous system there are specialized cells, including nerve cells, also known as neurons. Neurons are those little gems that serve as the rapid-fire communication system, which send signals to other cells in the body to get things done.

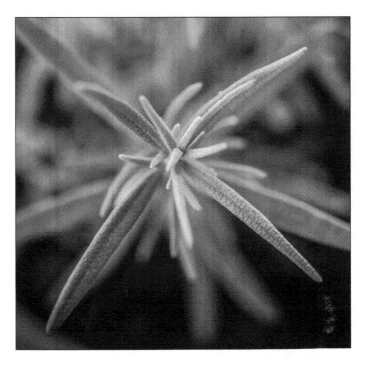

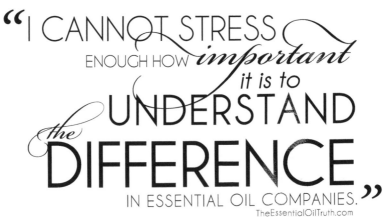

"I CANNOT STRESS ENOUGH HOW *important* it is to UNDERSTAND *the* DIFFERENCE IN ESSENTIAL OIL COMPANIES."

Neurological disorders, toxicity, genetic defects, memory loss, vision loss, hearing loss or tinnitus, dizziness, infection, disease, old age, cognitive loss, speech impairments, plus a whole host of ailments can all stem from a breakdown of the nervous system. A healthy nervous system is paramount to a healthy body. It is important to support the health and wellness of the nervous system and essential oils are a great way to do just that.

Essential oils that may help support the nervous system:
Basil, Bergamot, Black Pepper, Cedarwood, Cinnamon Bark, Copaiba, Cypress, Eucalyptus, Frankincense, Geranium, Ginger, Grapefruit, Helichrysum, Juniper, Lemon, Lemongrass, Lavender, Nutmeg, Peppermint, Ravintsara, Roman Chamomile, Spearmint, Spruce, Valerian, Vetiver

To help support your nervous system on a daily basis, consider using Frankincense on the back of your neck just below your skull. You may also consider applying Helichrysum as well.

Another great way to help rid the spinal chord of toxins is to have several high detoxifying essential oils rubbed along your back on either side of your spine. You can start by placing some carrier oil along your spine and then apply such oils as Oregano, Basil, Marjoram, Peppermint, Frankincense, or any other oils you know will enhance the area you would like support with.

Using over-the-counter essential oils or ones that you cannot verify as fully pure, organic essential oils could do more harm than good. I cannot stress enough how important it is to understand the difference in essential oil companies, especially if you try to undertake placing essential oils directly on your spine.

Lesson #38
ESSENTIAL OILS & THE REPRODUCTIVE SYSTEM

The reproduction system encompasses our sex organs as well as our hormones and pheromones. It also involves the process of menstruation, fertilization, gestation, labor and delivery, and nursing. Men have two jobs; to make sperm and get it to the right place. Women have three jobs; to make eggs and then get them fertilized, but also to provide a safe gestational period for the baby before it is born. A healthy reproductive system in both male and female partners who wish to create another human is important to the health of the gestating mom and the growing and developing child.

Essential oils help support the reproductive system in many ways. One thing you may be starting to understand is how interconnected all our systems are. Simply supporting the circulatory, lymphatic, nervous, endocrine, and limbic systems can make all the difference in the world for the reproductive system.

Proper circulation will help support healthy blood flow to the necessary areas. Proper waste management and immune support through our lymph create a healthful environment in gestational development. The nervous system must be firing and communicating well to also create a healthful environment. The endocrine must supply the necessary hormones and enzymes needed for reproduction. Lastly, the limbic system (through aromatherapy) may help enhance our mood and sexual drive, as well as encourage release of emotional trauma and mental blocks.

Essential oils that support the reproductive system:

Menstruation: Lavender, Ginger, Cypress, Marjoram, Roman Chamomile, Clary Sage

Sexual Drive: Orange, Ylang ylang, Jasmine, Peppermint, Rose, Sandalwood, Goldenrod, Cypress

Fertility: Geranium, Ylang ylang, Clary Sage

Pregnancy: Peppermint (aromatically only), Lavender, Ginger, Ylang ylang

Nursing: Roman Chamomile, Lavender, Tangerine, Basil, Clary Sage, Fennel

As mentioned in lesson #29, the introduction to the body systems, this list is not exhaustive. Please also refer to the other lessons on the body systems, as well as lesson #23 on Pregnancy. These essential oils may be used aromatically, topically, and internally in some cases. Please double check with the label for each individual bottle for proper use.

*L*esson #39
ESSENTIAL OILS & THE RESPIRATORY SYSTEM

The respiratory system is a set of specific organs that process and exchange oxygen for carbon dioxide. We inhale oxygen into our lungs, it processes the oxygen, and through a gas exchange, we exhale carbon dioxide. This process oxygenates the blood while removing metabolic waste, including carbon dioxide, from the circulatory system. When the respiratory system is not at optimal health, other systems are affected such as the immunity, circulatory, lymphatic, and endocrine through metabolic function. Essential oils can greatly enhance the health and wellness of the respiratory system through aromatherapy. By simply breathing in essential oil molecules we are creating a more healthful air quality. Not only does the simplicity of smelling an essential oil support the health of our overall respiratory system, but also diffusing them into the air will raise the amount of negative ions in the room.

When you are near a body of water such as an ocean, lake, waterfall, or even a pool, your body will feel more energized. Water creates an environment that contains more negative ions, and places lacking water, or places with an abundance of technology, such as the workplace or larger cities will have more positive ions. Negative ions help create a more positive, calming mood. Denise Mann, on WebMD.com states, "Once they reach our bloodstream, negative ions are believed to produce biochemical reactions that increase levels of the mood chemical serotonin, helping to alleviate depression, relieve stress, and boost our daytime energy."

Positive ions are why people are more irritable before a storm, and usually everyone is calm and collected just after a storm. Another interesting fact to note is all the strange behavior that seems to happen around a full moon. Science can explain it plainly because there is an increase of positive ion ratios when there is a full moon. There are times that we may need an increase in positive ions when we live in areas that are abundant in negative ions such as near the ocean or a waterfall. Positive ions are responsible for stimulating the sympathetic nervous system, our fight or flight responses. Essential oils such as Clove, Cypress, Eucalyptus, Frankincense, Rosemary, Thyme, and Ylang ylang, to name a few, will ionize positively when diffused.

EMR Labs, LLC states, "Negative ions are exceedingly beneficial for a person's metabolism as a means of enhancing human behavior. They act in a complex mechanism to bring about hormone and biochemical reactions in the body and brain. It is impossible to get an overdose of negative ions, which act like pure water in washing away dirty poisons. Generally, the more negative ions you are exposed to, the better and more uplifted you feel. Positive ions or the lack of negative ions may cause serotonin hyper-function syndrome or "irritation syndrome" involves sleeplessness, irritability, tension, migraine, nausea, heart palpitations, hot flashes with sweating or chills, tremors and dizziness. The elderly become depressed, apathetic and extremely fatigued."

The following chart lists the average ions present in the air per 1 cubic centimeter as stated by EMR Labs, LLC.

AVERAGE IONS PER 1 CM³		
LOCATION	NEGATIVE	POSITIVE
Waterfalls	100,000+	
Clean mountain air	2,000	2,500
Normal air on land	1,500	1,800
Air just before a storm	750	2,500
Air just after a storm	2,500	750
Office workspace with normal technology	150	200
Inside car with windows rolled up while driving	50	150

The respiratory system can greatly enhance our overall mood health simply by diffusing essential oils into the air using a cold-water, ultrasonic, ionizing, humidifying diffuser. Dr. Vanessa Perez, Ph.D. and Managing Scientist at

Exponent, Inc. states in her study on air ions and mood outcomes in January 2013, "Negative air ionization was associated with lower depression scores particularly at the highest exposure level."

Adding specific oils can help increase the negative ionizing affects such as Bergamot, Cedarwood, Citronella, Eucalyptus, Grapefruit, Lavender, Lemon, Lemongrass, Mandarin, Orange, and Sandalwood. Adding these oils to your diffuser does not mean, however, that they will energize you. Negative ions work beneficially for you during the day and night. During the day, they will enhance your mood and allow for a general sense of well-being. During the night, they will produce a calm environment, free of restlessness.

While negative ions are something to consider when looking at your respiratory system for mood enhancing health, generally speaking, there have been no findings that negative ions are physically beneficial for your actual respiratory system. That is where essential oils come in. Eucalyptus essential oil is one of the most commonly used oils to support the respiratory system. Breathing it in is the obvious usage choice, however placing a drop on your jugular notch, which is the hollow area between your collarbones at the base of your throat, works well too.

Another commonly used essential oil is Peppermint. When breathed in, it gives you an open feeling in your lungs. This essential oil is great to ingest as long as you are using an ingestible Peppermint essential oil. Place about 3-4 drops in an empty capsule, top off with a carrier oil, and swallow. Doing this once or twice a day will support a more healthful respiratory system.

Essential oils that support the respiratory system:
Bergamot, Clove, Cinnamon Bark, Cinnamon Leaf, Eucalyptus, Fennel, Fir, Frankincense, Helichrysum, Hyssop, Lavender, Ledum, Lemon, Lemongrass, Marjoram, Oregano, Peppermint, Ravintsara, Sage, Spearmint, Tea Tree

Rubbing essential oils on your chest, lymph nodes, sinus areas, and inhaling them in directly or through the use of a diffuser encourages a more healthful respiratory function. Daily use of respiratory support essential oils is recommended, especially when the seasons change. Seasonal changes usually bring changes in air quality and temperature. Be prepared by checking weather patterns and being aware of when the seasons change, and don't leave home without your trusted respiratory support essential oils.

esson #40

ESSENTIAL OILS & THE SKELETAL SYSTEM

The skeletal system is a complex network of bones, tendons, ligaments, and cartilage. An adult human body consists of 206 bones, 52 of which are found just in the feet. Bones are a living organism and thrive because of the circulatory and nervous system. They are surrounded by blood vessels and nerves, and are made of a dense outer layer and a spongy secondary layer. Some bones contain bone marrow, which produces red blood cells. Bone marrow supports the immune system and is an important part of the lymphatic system. Teeth are also part of the skeletal system, and play an important part in the digestive system, as well as the skeletal system.

Essential oils help in many areas of the skeletal system to support healthful function. The use of Tea Tree and Lemon essential oils are a great way to care for your teeth. I often get asked, "Why Lemon? Isn't that high in acid?" Lemon essential oil contains no acid. It is pH neutral, but is a great brightening agent. Tea Tree essential oil supports healthy gums and, in turn, supports healthy teeth. Wintergreen is a natural osteo support essential oil and is a perfect choice to daily place diluted on the skin directly over bone areas you want to enhance. A wonderful synergy would be equal parts of Wintergreen, Helichrysum, and Clove.

Essential oils that support the skeletal system:

Tendons and Ligaments: Helichrysum, Lemongrass

Cartilage: Peppermint, Sandalwood, White Fir

Bones: Clove, Cypress, Fennel, Fir, Geranium, Hyssop, Lemon, Oregano, Peppermint, Pine, Rosemary, Spruce, Thyme, Wintergreen

The best way to help support a healthy skeletal system is to rub specific essential oils on the location of need, as well as to embark upon a daily internal regimen of specific consumable essential oils. Research each essential oil and what their specific properties are so you know how to best support your skeletal system.

*L*esson #41
ESSENTIAL OILS & THE RENAL SYSTEM
(urinary)

The renal system is also called the urinary system. It is comprised of the bladder, kidneys, ureters (which transfer urine from the kidneys to the bladder), and urethra. The renal system has several functions. It eliminates waste, regulates blood pressure, blood volume, and blood pH, and it regulates the electrolyte and metabolite levels. Blood filters through the kidney to create urine. It is then stored in the bladder until it is released through urination.

Essential oils that support the renal system:

Bergamot, Copaiba, Eucalyptus, Geranium, Goldenrod, Hyssop, Juniper, Lavender, Ledum, Lemon, Lemongrass, Myrtle, Oregano, Pine, Rosemary, Sandalwood, Thyme

Drinking essential oil-infused water is a great way to help support a healthy renal system. Based on your needs, you may use any of the above listed oils. You may also rub essential oils over your lower abdomen and back, and even your pubic area. When it is desired to increase the healthy function of the urethra, many women find it helpful to use a retention tampon dipped in a mixture of 2 tablespoons of Olive oil with 3-10 drops of specific essential oils. With this method, dilution is the key.

Most of us do not consume enough water and end up with a poorly functioning renal system. It is recommended that we drink half our body weight in ounces each day. That means if you weigh 150 pounds you should be drinking 75 ounces a day. Your urine should be a clear, pale-yellow color. If it is yellow or has a pungent odor, you are not drinking enough water or you are simply taxing your liver by taking too many man-made supplements that are going right down the drain.

Utilizing essential oils in your daily intake of water not only makes it taste better, like an amazing spa water, but it also helps to flush your system based on the specific oils you use. As I have said throughout this book, please make certain you are only using FDA approved, ingestible essential oils.

*L*esson #42
ESSENTIAL OILS FOR HOME USE

For most of us our home is where we spend 1/3 of our entire lives, if not more. With that in mind, consider the air quality in your home. When was the last time you had your furnace cleaned? Oddly most homeowners and even renters will go years, if not decades, not even knowing that the air quality in their home is compromised, simply because of a dirty furnace. While getting a good furnace cleaning every other year or so is important for the air quality of your home, where do essential oils come in?

The air filters are part of the air system in our homes and those should be changed out every 3-4 months, or at least once a year. The best thing you can do to improve the air quality in your home is to drop 20 drops of Tea Tree essential oil (or other favorite oil) all over a new air filter before you install it. Then, run the air for about an hour. Your whole home will smell wonderful and will be filled with the cleansing scent of the essential oil you used. It becomes a huge "whole home" diffuser. If you have easy access to your air filter consider dropping essential oils on your filter once a week.

I also recommend that you purchase an ionizing, ultrasonic room diffuser for every major room in your home. Consider one for each bedroom to diffuse essential oils at night, in order to promote a more restful sleep. You may want to have another one for your home office to promote alertness and energy while on your computer or reading. You may also wish to have one in your living area, one in your kitchen, and one in each of your main bathrooms. There are even such things as card diffusers and diffuser jewelry.

Essential oils also have the ability to naturally clean surfaces without the use of harsh and harmful chemical cleaning agents. Lemon has the wonderful ability to cut through grime and acts as a swift degreaser on pots and pans, as well as removes sticker residue. Essential oils are even great for when your child decides to use your living room wall as an art canvas for their crayon masterpiece. There are so many other uses for the home; the list is endless. Here is a short list to give you an idea of the array of areas you may use essential oils: Linen spray, bath and tile cleaner, dog bed freshener, laundry stains, dryer sheet enhancer, lawn and garden support, car freshener, car degreaser, floor cleaner, and surface cleaner.

Essential oils that may be used in the home:

> *Cleaning:* Lemon, Tea Tree, Clove, Cinnamon Bark, Peppermint, Fir, Spruce.

> *Nighttime diffuser:* Lavender, Cedarwood, Frankincense, Vetiver, Valerian, Roman Chamomile, Geranium, Rose, Ylang ylang, or any combination.

> *Daytime diffuser:* Lavender, Vetiver, Orange, Lemon, Grapefruit or any citrus essential oil, Peppermint, Rosemary, Tea Tree or any combination.

> *Garden:* Lavender, Peppermint, Lemon, Basil, Cinnamon Bark, Sage, Thyme. (Place a few drops of desired essential oil in a glass spray bottle and spray around your yard.)

For personal use, consider using essential oils for your toothpaste, underarm and foot odor support, mouthwash, nail hardener, scalp freshener, body serum, face serum, hair support, lip balm, hand and body wash, beard balm, aftershave, as well as many other uses.

Cold-water diffuser recipes are fun to create to find the perfect seasonal scents for your home. You can find 40 diffuser recipes in the book, "French Aromatherapy: Essential Oil Recipes and Usage Guide". Here are a few to get you started for each season change.

Cold-water Diffuser Recipes:
Mix synergy by adding 10 times the below amount in a clean bottle, then drip 6 drops of your synergy into a full 300-400mL water basin in your cold-water diffuser.

Seasonal: Spring – 4 drops Orange and 2 drops Peppermint

Seasonal: Summer – 3 drops each Ylang ylang and Bergamot

Seasonal: Fall – 4 drops Orange and 2 drops Cinnamon Bark

Seasonal: Winter – 3 drops Orange, 2 drops Spruce, 1 drop each Fir, Clove, and Cinnamon Bark

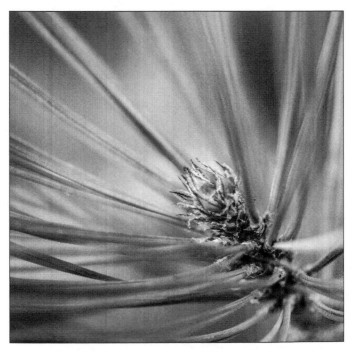

" TO BE CONSIDERED TRULY
organic
LAND SHOULD BE FREE OF ALL
CHEMICALS
FOR A MINIMUM OF
50 *Years* "

TheEssentialOilTruth.com

Lesson #43
ESSENTIAL OILS & LAND

Did you know that for land to be considered organic it must be chemical-free, meaning all farming practices are to use chemical-free seeds, water, fertilizer, pesticides, germicides, and harvest methods for at least 7 years? That amount of time is the regulatory standard in place however, to be considered truly organic, land should be free of all chemical use including run-off from other surrounding farms for a minimum of 50 years.

When choosing a company for your essential oils it is imperative that you ask if the land that their plants are grown on is organic and if so for how many years? If they do not know, or are unable to answer, then, in most cases, they are not organic. If they say they are organic but cannot answer how many years it is most likely the 7-year mark.

Would that matter to you if it were 7 years or 50? That is up to you. Personally I would rather get my essential oils from a company that is able to source their material from truly organic-organic. It is sad that there is even such a need to say "organic-organic". Much like finding "pure-pure" essential oil, it is something we need to at least be aware of to make an informed decision on the products we put on and in our bodies.

Lesson #44
ESSENTIAL OILS & SEED SELECTION

It may not be something you have ever considered before, but think about it; a bad egg will produce a bad chicken, a less than perfect embryo will produce a deformed or disabled human, just like a less than perfect seed will produce inferior plant material.

When I was considering having a baby, you better believe I was in full-blown research mode. Talk about being obsessed. I had to figure out all the information and the "right way" to embark on the oh-so-important path of making another human. This was serious stuff. An interesting analogy I was told had to do with being infertile, which thankfully we were not, however it is a good example to understand why seed selection is so important.

When you get checked for infertility they basically determine if the female has eggs and if the male has sperm. They check the male out a little more by finding out how many sperm are in an ejaculation as well as if they are good swimmers. That's it. They do not check to see if the eggs or the sperm are good specimens or even DNA viable. It was explained like this: a shipping company ships millions of packages. While there are lots of packages (sperm), and they all, hopefully get to their destination (the egg), there is no way that shipping company knows what is in each package. There could be crystal glass vases that are in perfect condition, or there could be crystal glass vases that are all shattered.

The beauty of our bodies is that if a sperm and egg find each other, once the growth process begins if, in any way, the egg/sperm combo DNA is lacking, in most cases our bodies will simply miscarry. It is a natural "survival of the fittest" progression. When it comes to seed selection and harvesting, sure you could use any purchased seed, even a GMO (genetically modified organism) seed, and guess what? The plant material used for essential oil extraction will produce vastly different constituents that are often times undesirable.

Consider the GMO seed for a moment. One of the very reasons essential oils are so powerful is because their constituents are continually and consistently changing with each new crop. If a company is using a seed that was created for consistency, quantity, growth speed, and reliability (the main reasons most GMOs are created) then you will loose a very desirable component of the power of essential oils and their ability to adapt with us and for us.

How, then, should a company select their seeds? The absolute best way is from their choicest crop from the year prior. This is assuming they used the most desirable farming methods. Once again, this is something you need to consider when choosing your essential oil company.

Lesson #45
ESSENTIAL OILS & CULTIVATION

Cultivation covers everything from soil preparation, seeding, fertilization, watering, including irrigation and rain, sun exposure, climate, air quality, pest control and bacteria control, to harvest methods and timing. As you can imagine, each step of the process is critical to creating the most choice plant materials to use for essential oil production.

This is something most people don't consider or even know they should consider. While all are important, one area that is interesting is the company's ability to determine the exact right time to harvest their crops. The maturity of the plant is paramount to producing the right constituents of an essential oil. We understand that a baby should be born at just the right time just like picking an apple from a tree when it is ripe has a far greater nutrient value than one picked two weeks before ripening, as is the case with most store-bought produce.

The cultivation process is an area of consideration simply because it determines the constituent value and usefulness of the essential oil that it creates. While most areas of the cultivation process can be controlled there are a few areas that are completely out of human control such as sun exposure, too much rain, and air quality from wind patterns.
While reputable farmers do all they can to promote quality growth, occasionally what is called an "act of God" occurs that is outside of their control. When this happens, why should you be concerned?

Most essential oil plant life growers are more concerned with bottom line sales and production than the actual constituents. There is an exact right time of day that a plant should be harvested. There is a specific amount of time that plant life should "rest" after harvest to obtain the highest quality of essential oils.

When things go wrong, either inside or outside of the control of the farmers it is important to know how your oil company deals with such potential mistakes. Do they test the oil and buy it if it is in range of their quality? If it is not in range of their quality and they do not buy it, do they know if the grower allows someone else to buy it? If they do, does your company still work with that company knowing that an inferior product is being sold to the highest bidder? Is that unethical to you? These are all questions you need to answer. If you do not care, then be prepared to get oils that should essentially be dumped down the drain.

Ethically speaking, when something goes wrong in the production and cultivation of plant life and an oil is created that is sub-par, the oil should be dumped. Literally. Dumped. It should not go to market. Too often I have called companies to ask what they do with oils that do not pass inspection and they say they resell it.

One company I spoke with in my quest for the best essential oils said that they "do the best they can with testing" and they only know it is a bad oil when too many people complain. They then went on to say that when that happens, they recall that oil. They tried to re-assure me by stating it rarely happens. Rarely happens? It should not happen at all. If an oil tests below standards, it should be dumped. Period. Even if the dumping of that oil is a million dollar mistake. That may sound harsh, but the reality is, we rely on the companies we use to sell us products in keeping with their promises. More on this topic will be discussed in Lesson 48 on testing.

Lesson #46
ESSENTIAL OILS & EXTRACTION

There are several methods of essential oil extraction, however, the top two methods of extraction of therapeutic grade essential oils are steam distillation and cold press, also known as expression. We covered the most important aspects of extraction of essential oils via steam distillation in lessons 16-18.

To re-cap, steam distillation is the method used to extract the essential oil from plant material using a low temperature, low or no pressure process. Plant material is placed on a grate that is hovering over the top of boiling water. The steam from the water passes through the plant material and up into a collection tube, where the steam carrying the tiny volatile essential oil molecules collects and forms back into water, then travels down the tube and separates into the essential oil and water distillate, also known as fragrant water, or hydrosol.

The top quality essential oils are extracted using very low heat and no pressure to ensure the constituents are not compromised. Constituents boil at different rates and the most volatile ones boil first. The more fragrant and less therapeutic constituents boil last and are sometimes unnecessary, however most all oil companies offer essential oils containing as many of the constituents as possible based on the cost to produce them. The fact of the matter is, most companies buy oils from brokers and have no idea that the oils themselves have simply been processed incorrectly, and therefore, have less therapeutic qualities. While these essential oils may still be good quality oils, they may be less strong than oils that were distilled correctly.

Another commonly used form of extraction is cold pressing, which is also referred to as expression. This method is often used in extracting essential oils from the rinds of citrus fruits such as Lemon, Orange, Bergamot, and others. It is also used to extract carrier type oils like Olive oil, Grapeseed oil, and Coconut oil. Cold pressing involves hydraulic pressure on the rinds of citrus and other materials like seeds, grains, and nuts. It is commonly done at room temperature however some involve very low temperature to get the desired results. The best quality is virgin or first press oils, which indicate they are simply pressed; no solvent, heat, or any other chemical interaction was involved.

Carrier oils like Olive oil that are extra-virgin are ones that are considered to be the most pure, meaning there is no refining or chemicals involved in the process of making it. You can test your Olive oil by placing it in the refrigerator. If the oil turns to a crystalline form, it is most likely an extra-virgin Olive oil. If it forms a solid block, it is most likely refined, possibly using chemicals. Companies may still be permitted to call it virgin Olive oil because a small amount of virgin Olive oil is contained in the overall oil.

A truly pure cold pressed essential oil will be extracted at room temperature. Higher temperatures will yield higher batch quantities of oils with altered constituents. The best cold pressed essential oils are those done without any heat. However, because the essential oil labeling in the US is not regulated there is no way of knowing if heat was applied during the cold press process.

The easiest way to tell if you have an "extra-virgin" cold pressed essential oil (there is no actual term used in the industry, but for sake of illustration and understanding I am using the term "extra-virgin" in quotes), you can place a drop of Lemon essential oil from several different companies onto a Styrofoam cup. You will see plainly which oil is more potent; however, that is not only because of how it was pressed, but also how it was cultivated from start to finish. To truly know the quality of your oil, you must also know the quality of the land, seed selection, and cultivation as discussed in Lessons 43-45.

*L*esson #47
ESSENTIAL OILS & TESTING

Any high quality product should go through testing and quality control to ensure each batch of that product is up to the standards the company has set forth. Gas chromatography paired with the use of mass spectroscopy (referred to as GC/MS) can help to ensure general range. However, there is no actual standardization of essential oils, simply because nature cannot be standardized. This type of testing requires a master in the art of essential oil analysis to interpret the findings from the GC/MS tests.

Other tests included alongside a CG/MS would be a flame ionization detector (FID) and isotope ratio (IR). These would start with the CG then move to the FID and IR and end with the MS to analyze the findings. Several other tests should also include specific gravity, refractive index, flash point (combustibility), optical rotation, and microbial testing. When a lab offers all of these test, it is a good indicator that they are a good lab, but may not be entirely conclusive based on the chemical profiles that lab has on file from past tests.

There is a European standard for the actual chemical profiles and constituents that should be present in essential oils of the highest standard. This standard is based on the International Standards Organization (ISO) and the Association French Normalization Organization Regulation (AFNOR). Because not all essential oils companies use this standard, testing can become subjective, especially when their tests are only performed in-house. It is far better to buy your essential oils from a company that does a three-pronged testing procedure using one or more standardization methods, including AFNOR.

The main issue with getting an essential oil analyzed is what company you are testing your oil through. There is a litmus test with every lab. That litmus test is their library. The library is the data stored from thousands upon thousands of past tests. The quality of the lab can only be determined by the quality and extensiveness of the library that the lab uses. While the average person could hire a smaller, less experienced lab to test an oil for a mere $140-200, if you conduct a full set of tests at a lab that historically and physically has the data in their library to qualify and analyze that specific essential oil, the price tag ranges from $800 to $1,000. Historically, you would need to look at a company's track record. It would not make sense for a company to use synthetics in a batch of essential oils when they often take a popular essential oil off the market because of a sub-par batch.

In-house testing is important for the company to know that what they are placing in the hands of their customers is what they promised. The second method would be third party testing, where an outside company verifies that the product is, in fact, what the company states it is. Third party testing can be tricky to find in an essential oil company because it is expensive. A company should also perform side-by-side comparisons between their product and other essential oils of the same noted quality, to ensure the constituents in their oil is on par or exceeds that of other brands. This third check is also something most companies do not perform because of the expense involved.

With any essential oil company, we trust that the information and guarantees they give us about their products are true and reliable. Sadly, this is not the case with many companies. They may not know 100% if the oil they get from a supplier is pure, because the majority of companies obtain their essential oils from third party suppliers. These suppliers may put additives in their oils to make them have a more desirable aroma. Such is the case with Ethyl Vanillin, which is a strong synthetic fragrant food additive often found in very reputable essential oils that are touted as pure. While these companies may do everything to test for purity, the machines they typically use are unable to test for anything above 0.1% of any given constituent. In several instances, third party testing found 0.07% of this Ethyl Vanillin in essential oils from two separate companies.

Further testing confirmed that the oils were exactly the same in constituent makeup, which indicated that both companies purchased from the same

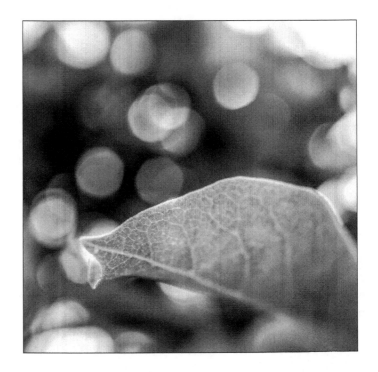

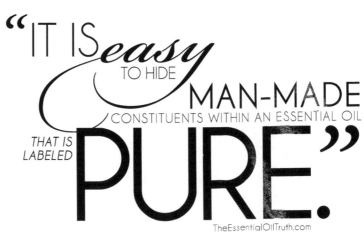

"IT IS *easy* TO HIDE MAN-MADE CONSTITUENTS WITHIN AN ESSENTIAL OIL THAT IS LABELED PURE."

supplier. There were counter tests done on the same batch of oils from another chemist who stated, emphatically, that the original test was somehow misread or tainted and that the oils are, in fact, pure, without any trace of synthetic additives. However, based on further research into the companies in question, and the person conducting the counter test, there is a conflict of interest and therefore, to trust the counter test would be a lack of good judgment. The first test is also not trustworthy because the investigation was not standardized, based on all the information noted on the subject. This is why it is important to get third party testing from someone without any monetary stake in the matter. While this issue is still in dispute, it makes us, the consumers wary of any and all oils when we don't personally have access to a million dollar gas chromatography machine.

This all can be extremely frustrating for the average essential oil user. While I understand this may seem like hype, and this book is not about hype, I felt it necessary to talk about the ethyl vanillin scandal because it is indicative of the world we live in. The company who purchased the essential oil did everything they could to test the oils, and to the best of their knowledge they were, in fact, pure. It just goes to show you that due to the very small size of essential oil constituents, along with the extremely intense fragrant properties of some synthetic substitutes, it is easy to hide man-made chemical constituents within an essential oil that is labeled "pure." Asking your essential oils company how they perform all evaluations and which tests they use, finding out if they do third party testing on their oils, as well as side-by-side comparisons of their oils vs. their competition may make all the difference in your ability to trust your essential oil provider.

Lesson #48
ESSENTIAL OILS & PRODUCT PACKAGING

Most companies purchase their essential oils from suppliers all over the world. When oils come out of the separators from the distilleries they will then go into a container to be transferred to the plant for bottling. Depending on where the oils are coming from, sometimes across the globe, there is no way of knowing if the container used was glass, stainless steel, or some other container that may have caused contamination.

Also, can you be sure there was no excessive heat during the summer months in the cargo unit when the essential oils were being transferred? Assuming they came to the lab intact, were decanted and filtered, and then were tested for purity and constituent potency, they will then carry them via secondary smaller containers to the bottling labs. Again, these containers must be stainless steel or glass. Typically they are stainless steel. Once they arrive at the bottling lab, they will go into the final decanters, which should be stainless steel, and finally into an amber or dark colored glass essential oil bottle.

Most companies follow standard bottling and packaging practices. The only concern would be when companies are sent oils from their third party suppliers that are contaminated *after* testing or in some cases labeled incorrectly. Human error happens all the time, so it is important to use a company that owns up to its mistakes if and when one is made.

It is also important to consider what procedures are put in place to keep errors from happening. One of the best questions you can ask your oils company when it comes to the full process of production, from cultivation to packaging, is if you can visit their farms, labs, and packaging plants. Some companies will say, "yes" to their packaging plants, however most oils companies do not allow touring of their farms because they do not own them or do not have the ability to allow consumers to tour their third party farms.

There are several companies that do own their own farms and you are able to visit and tour them all over the globe; from small production nunneries in Europe that produce boutique quality essential oils to large corporate companies that produce mass quantity. All you need to do is ask to know if your oils company allows you to tour their entire process. Visiting an essential oil farm, distillery, and production plant is one of the most educational and eye-opening adventures you can take. I highly recommend creating a holiday with you and your family as soon as possible. If you are an essential oil lover, or an aspiring essential oil lover, this profound experience will put you over the top.

FINAL THOUGHTS
ENCOURAGEMENT FROM JEN

It is my prayer that this book will help you become a more informed and confident essential oil user. When I first started using essential oils in 2007, I never realized just how incredible those small bottles were until, little by little, I used each one, and little by little became a true believer in their beautiful power.

It is hard to understand why people willingly eat powdered donuts, drink their chemically-laden coffee and diet sodas, and eat anything that is packaged in a box simply because the "powers-that-be" have told us we can eat it. Yet the moment I share a bottle of lavender essential oil with them, a product straight from nature, they shake their head, throw up their hands and tell me they need to research it before they would even *consider* using it. It is baffling, however, it is also the reason I wrote this book for you. There is so much hype and false information floating around regarding essential oils as well as straight up fear-inducing tactics to get people to question the safety of oils. There is good reason for this fear, simply because of the bastardizations of the essential oil industry.

These questionable companies are producing their essential oils quicker and cheaper by using constituent-depleting cultivation and extraction methods and many are adding fillers and other harmful chemicals making them essentially poison. It is no wonder the essential oil industry has become scary terrain to navigate. If, for any reason, you are still confused, I encourage you to read this book again. When I was a college professor for many years at College of the Canyons and Art Center College of Design I had the distinct pleasure of helping students learn complicated and technical information on advanced photography techniques as well as book publishing and construction. In those classes my students were always thankful for the continual repeating of information.

What I learned early on in my teaching career is that I could be lecturing on a topic, state very clearly that topic, and then a student would ask me a question that I just answered 5 minutes prior. While other students would roll their eyes, I would simply answer their question as if it was the first time I ever explained it, and it was their first time ever hearing the information. I would not stop

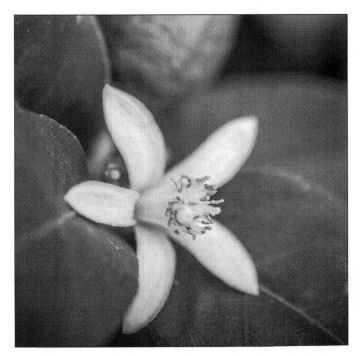

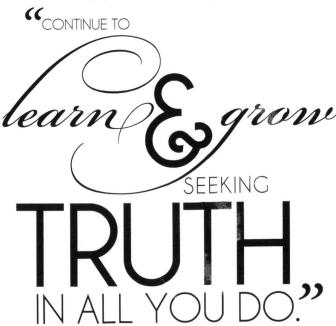

"CONTINUE TO *learn & grow* SEEKING

TRUTH
IN ALL YOU DO."

TheEssentialOilTruth.com

explaining or teaching until I saw the light go on in their eyes; that "a-ha" moment that every teacher looks for in his or her student's face.

Several students over the years questioned why I was so patient with those students who were seemingly daft. The simple answer; I understood not only that the information I was teaching was complicated, but it was also a lot of information. When there is a lot to take in, often our minds will process one section of information only to bypass the next section, even if we are reading it or being told it. It is as if our cognitive brain never heard or read the information.

For that simple reason I encourage you to re-read this book as many times as it takes for your brain to take it all in. It is a lot. Mark up the pages. Put questions in the margins. Dog-ear pages you want to return to. Study it and share it. I want to get essential oils into every home and every life. Not just any oils though, the right oils. This requires you to do your homework on the current company you use. Ask questions. Push. Find out. It is the only way to ensure purity and quality in the essential oils you use.

You matter to me. Really. You do. I do not look at you as a person, but a soul. You are created by God and in the image of God and for that simple, yet profound reason, I was compelled to write this book. If you still have questions you are more than welcome to contact me. It would be my honor to help you on your journey. A friend who uses oils may have given you this book. Talk to them. Ask them questions. Drill them for information. See what their company does and where they stack up compared to the information in this book. Then, when you are ready, jump in with both feet. Don't put it off. God created the plants to help us. Here is a verse in the Old Testament that you may have not considered. It is found in Ezekiel speaking of the New Jerusalem and was also later written in Revelation 22:2.

Ezekiel 47:12 ESV states, "And on the banks, on both sides of the river, there will grow all kinds of trees for food. Their leaves will not wither, nor their fruit fail, but they will bear fresh fruit every month, because the water for them flows from the sanctuary. Their fruit will be for food, and their leaves for healing." Their leaves are for healing! Meaning in the future. What a beautiful thing to consider as God's blessing for us. I wish you all the best on your path to better understanding of essential oils. With the ever-changing world we live in, I encourage you to continue to learn and grow seeking truth in all you do. Many blessings and abundant "life upon life" is my hope and prayer for you and your loved ones!

~ Jen

RESOURCES

Internet

General websites with multiple page reference use.
www.aromaticstudies.com
www.resourcegate.net
www.wikipedia.org
www.naha.org
www.alliance-aromatherapists.org
www.aromatherapycouncil.org
www.fao.org
www.fda.gov
www.cdc.gov
www.ncbi.nlm.nih.gov
www.roberttisserand.com
www.seedtoseal.com

Specific webpage references

http://missionscience.nasa.gov/ems/TourOfEMS_Booklet_Web.pdf
http://www.coherentresources.com/bt3_monitor
http://tainio.com/index.php?pageControl=about
http://www.coherentresources.com/bt3_monitor
http://www.royal-rife.com/
http://jjm.ajums.ac.ir/_jjm/documents/10-14HRG.pdf
http://www.ncbi.nlm.nih.gov/pubmed/26172328
http://www.ncbi.nlm.nih.gov/pmc/articles/PMC3796379/
http://www.abc.net.au/science/articles/2003/11/10/981339.htm
http://healthimpactnews.com/2013/why-essential-oils-heal-and-drugs-dont/#sthash.oL0HxH99.dp
http://orgchem.colorado.edu/Technique/Procedures/Distillation/Distillation.html
http://www.chem.umass.edu/~samal/269/distill.pdf
http://umm.edu/health/medical/altmed/treatment/aromatherapy
http://healthimpactnews.com/2014/fda-targets-essentials-oils-see-eos-as-threat-to-new-ebola-drug
http://www.cdc.gov/mmwr/preview/mmwrhtml/su6203a27.htm?s_
    cid=su6203a27_w#x2014;%20United%20States,%201999%E2%80%932010%3C/a%3E
http://www.cdc.gov/drugoverdose/index.html
http://www.atsdr.cdc.gov/substances/toxsubstance.asp?toxid=27
http://www2.estrellamountain.edu/faculty/farabee/BIOBK/BioBookNERV.html
http://www.faqs.org/health/Body-by-Design-V2/The-Nervous-System-Workings-how-the-
    nervous-system-functions.html http://medical-dictionary.thefreedictionary.com/sesquiterpen
http://roberttisserand.com/2012/08/book-review-the-chemistry-of-essential-oils-made-simple/
http://www.life.illinois.edu/ib/425/lecture19.html
http://jn.nutrition.org/content/129/3/775.long
http://www.ncbi.nlm.nih.gov/pubmed/16178774
http://animals.nationalgeographic.com/animals/fish/great-white-shark/
http://www.fao.org/docrep/V5350e/V5350e13.htm.
http://www.webmd.com/balance/features/negative-ions-create-positive-vibes
https://www.quantumbalancing.com/negative_ions.htm
http://www.ncbi.nlm.nih.gov/pubmed/23320516
http://www.livescience.com/22537-skeletal-system.html
http://www.fda.gov/Food/IngredientsPackagingLabeling/GRAS/default.htm

Books

Ames, G.R. and Matthews, W.S.A. (1968) The distillation of essential oils. Tropical Science.

Arctander, S. (1994). Perfume and Flavor Materials of Natural Origin. Carol Stream, Illinois: Allured Publishing Corporation.

Catty, S. (2001). Hydrosols: The Next Aromatherapy. Rochester, VT: Healing Arts Press.

Denny, E.F.K. (1991) Field Distillation for Herbaceous Oils. Lilydale, Tasmania.

Guba, R. (2002). The Modern Alchemy of Carbon Dioxide Extraction. International Journal of Aromatherapy.

Guenther, E. (1982). The Essential Oils. Melbourne, Fl: Krieger Publishing.

Life Science Publishing (2006) Essential Oils Desk Reference. Third Edition and Sixth Edition

Schnaubelt, K. (1999) Medical Aromatherapy. Frog Ltd, Berkeley, CA.

Schnaubelt, K. (2002). Biology of Essential Oils. San Rafael, CA: Terra Linda Scent.

Stewart, D. PhD (2003, 2014). Healing Oils of the Bible. Marble Hill, MO: Care Publications.

Tisserand, R. and Young, R. (2002, 20014) Essential Oil Safety: A Guide for Health Care Professionals. Second Edition. Churchill Livingstone Elsevier.

Food and Agriculture Organization of the United Nations (1995).

Williams, D. (1996). The Chemistry of Essential Oils. Dorset, England: Micelle Press.

Colleges

The School for Aromatic Studies

University of Colorado Boulder

UMass Amherst

University of Maryland, Medical Center

University of Illinois

Additional Resources

Get the App, THE EO BAR
Available for iOS and Android

EDUCATIONAL SITES

www.jenEssentials.com
www.youtube.com/c/jenosullivan
www.facebook.com/groups/jenessentials
www.facebook.com/groups/TheHumanBody
www.facebook.com/groups/IgniteAcademy

WORKSHOPS & COACHING

Jen teaches weekly workshops on essential oil use and health & wellness.
She is available for worldwide speaking engagements and workshops.
jen@jenosullivan.com

BOOKS AVAILABLE BY JEN

**For bulk purchasing of any of her books please go to
www.jenEssentials.com/books**

FRENCH AROMATHERAPY: ESSENTIAL OIL RECIPES & USAGE GUIDE
*The essential oil users guide to proper use and dosage using the French method
of Aromatherapy. Over 300 recipes along with several usage tips you may have
never considered before, this book is a must have for any library.*
Available on Amazon and at www.jenessentials.com

THE MARKETING INSOMNIAC
*The entrepreneur's go-to handbook on everything marketing, from how to
properly set up and use social media platforms such as Facebook, Instagram,
and Periscope, to other marketing tactics you may not have ever considered.*
Available on Amazon and www.MarketingInsomniac.com

Made in the USA
San Bernardino, CA
11 August 2016